QUICKCALC

MED DOSAGE CALCULATIONS

QUICKCALC
MED DOSAGE CALCULATIONS

Merrilee Tolhurst McDuffie

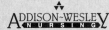
ADDISON-WESLEY
NURSING
A DIVISION OF
THE BENJAMIN/CUMMINGS PUBLISHING COMPANY, INC.

Redwood City, California • Menlo Park, California
Reading, Massachusetts • New York • Don Mills, Ontario
Wokingham, U.K. • Amsterdam • Bonn • Sydney • Singapore
Tokyo • Madrid • San Juan

Sponsoring Editor: Patricia L. Cleary
Developmental Editor: Mark F. Wales
Editorial Assistant: Megan Rundel
Senior Production Supervisor: Judith Hibbard
Outside Services Supervisor: Rani Cochran
Production Coordination: The Book Company
Text Design: Wendy Calmenson/The Book Company
Cover Supervisor: Yvo Riezebos
Cover Designer: Rodolphe Zehntner/Belmont Studios
Text and Cover Illustrator: Mary Ross
Copy Editor: Bonnie Kelsey
Senior Manufacturing Coordinator: Merry Free Osborn
Compositor: Jonathan Peck Typographers

Library of Congress Cataloging-in-Publication Data
McDuffie, Merrilee Tolhurst.
    QuickCalc : med dosage calculations / Merrilee Tolhurst McDuffie.
       p.   cm.
     ISBN 0-8053-1366-4
     1. Pharmaceutical arithmetic--Programmed instruction.   2. Nursing-
-Programmed instruction.   I. Title.
     [DNLM: 1. Drugs--administration & dosage--programmed instruction.
2. Drugs--administration & dosage--nurses' instruction.
3. Mathematics--programmed instruction.   4. Mathematics--nurses'
instruction.   QV 18 M478q 1994]
RS57.M34   1994
615'.14'0151--dc20
DNLM/DLC
for Library of Congress   93-39298
                                                   CIP

Care has been taken to confirm the accuracy of information presented in this book. The authors, editors, and publisher, however, cannot accept any responsibility for errors or omissions or for consequences from application of the information in this book and make no warranty, express or implied, with respect to its contents.

    The authors and publisher have exerted every effort to ensure that drug selections and dosages set forth in this text are in accord with current recommendations and practice at the time of publication. However, in view of ongoing research, changes in government regulations, and the constant flow of information relating to drug therapy and drug reactions, the reader is urged to check the package inserts of all drugs for any change in indications of dosage and for added warnings and precautions. This is particularly important when the recommended agent is a new and/or infrequently employed drug. Mention of a particular generic or brand name drug is not an endorsement, nor an implication that it is preferable to other named or unnamed agents.

ISBN 0-8053-1366-4
1 2 3 4 5 6 7 8 9 10—BAH 98 97 96 95 94

Addison-Wesley Nursing
A division of The Benjamin/Cummings Publishing Company, Inc.
390 Bridge Parkway
Redwood City, California 94065

Preface

QuickCalc is a programmed learning tool designed and written for students of nursing or allied health care professions who need to learn dosage calculation skills. Currently practicing professionals and those returning to the health care field also will find *QuickCalc* useful as a review of essential dosage calculation skills. This book can be used for self-directed learning or in a classroom setting.

How *QuickCalc* Works

QuickCalc introduces dosage calculation skills using a proven step-by-step technique that enables you to learn at your own pace. You will learn to calculate drug dosages using the "ratio-and-proportion" method—one of the safest and most popular techniques in use today. Ample practice opportunities allow you to assess how well you understand one skill or competency before you move on to the next. Here's what you'll learn:

We begin with your "road map" to *QuickCalc*. You'll learn how to follow the book's easy, programmed format for learning to make drug dosage calculations.

Section I: The first four chapters offer a quick review of essential number skills: Roman numerals, fractions, decimals, and solving for unknown amounts. A pretest at the start of this section will help you assess your need to study these skills. If you do well on this test, you can skip forward to Chapter 5.

Section II: Chapters 5 through 8 cover the three measurement systems you need to understand in order to read medication orders and calculate drug dosages: the metric system, the apothecary system, and the household system. You'll learn the basics of each system and how to convert dosage measurements from one system to another.

Section III: In Chapters 9 through 12 you'll learn how to calculate drug dosages for the most important oral and injectable medications. These chapters also cover skills such as reading medication orders and drug labels, and provide basic information about syringes.

Section IV: Chapters 13 and 14 tell you how to calculate the flow rate, dosage, and infusion time for solutions and drugs administered intravenously. You'll also learn how to modify medication dosages for infants and children.

Section V: The comprehensive exam in this section is formulated to assess your mastery of all the dosage calculation skills you will need to practice successfully as a nurse or health care professional.

Section VI: In Appendixes A through D you'll find some useful tools to help you interpret doctors' medication orders, convert between different systems of measurement, and modify drug dosages for infants and children. You will also find an illustrated overview of medication preparation forms.

Special Features of *QuickCalc*

- *QuickCalc* features the ratio-and-proportion method of dosage calculation—a method that's safe, easy to learn, and widely used.
- *QuickCalc*'s proven, interactive, programmed learning format will teach you one concept or skill at a time.
- You'll be able to practice on hundreds of **realistic** drug dosage calculation problems that feature the medications you'll encounter most frequently in practice.
- Unlike other books, *QuickCalc* shows you all the steps for solving **every** dosage calculation problem—not just the answers.
- *QuickCalc* teaches you to read and interpret actual drug labels.
- Important concepts and precautions are highlighted within special, easy-to-find boxes.

Calculating medication dosages safely is a fundamental part of your professional role in providing quality health care. Through *QuickCalc*, you will learn to perform this role effectively and confidently.

Reviewers

Patricia Fraser, MSN, CPNP
Hygiene, Colorado

Harold Hauser
Mt. Hood Community College
Gresham, Oregon

Ida Heath, RN
Peyton, Colorado

Kathy Halligan, MS, RN
University of Texas at Austin School of Nursing
Austin, Texas

Janet Joost, RN-C
Boulder Technical Education Center
Boulder, Colorado

Roselena Thorpe, RN, PhD
Community College of Allegheny County
Pittsburgh, Pennsylvania

Acknowledgments

I want to sincerely thank all my colleagues, reviewers, and students who have helped me craft this book. Special thanks go to the following people at Addison-Wesley Nursing: Mark McCormick, Project Editor, who guided and supported me during the planning of the book; Mark Wales, Developmental Editor, who encouraged me through an intense editing process; and Megan Rundel, Editorial Assistant, who assisted me through each step of the editorial process. Also, my thanks to Steve Tracy, Media Specialist at Boulder TEC, who was my liaison with many pharmaceutical companies. In addition, I gratefully acknowledge Janet Joost, BSN, RNC, and Patricia Frasier, MSN, CPNP, who expertly critiqued the intravenous therapy and pediatric dosage chapters.

I wish to acknowledge the pharmaceutical companies that granted me permission to reproduce the drug labels found within this book. They include:

- Abbott Laboratories
- Boehringer Ingelheim Pharmaceutical, Inc.
- Bristol-Myers Squibb
- Burroughs Wellcome Co.
- Eli Lilly and Company
- Geneva Pharmaceuticals, Inc.

- Marion Merrell Dow, Inc.
- Pfizer Inc.
- SmithKline Beecham
- The Upjohn Company

And finally, I want to specially thank my husband, Wayne, and son, Chad, for their patience, understanding, and support while I wrote, and wrote, and wrote.

Merrilee Tolhurst McDuffie

Contents

Section II: Systems of Measurement for Dosage Calculations

Section IV: Special Drug Dosage Calculations

Section V: Comprehensive Examination

Section VI: Tools

How to Use *QuickCalc*

QuickCalc is a programmed approach to learning basic drug dosage calculation skills. The advantage of a programmed approach is that it allows you to learn at your own pace and to receive immediate reinforcement about key concepts. Here's how *QuickCalc* works.

Chapter Outline, Objectives, and Introduction

At the start of every chapter in *QuickCalc*, you will find an outline of the basic topics and skills you need to master by the time you finish the chapter. To reinforce your goals, a list of learning objectives follows the outline. The chapter introduction provides a brief overview of essential background information or key concepts. After studying each of these features carefully, you can begin working through the "frames."

Programmed Learning Frames to Introduce Ideas and Skills

Each concept, skill, or competency in *QuickCalc* is introduced to you over a series of **frames**. Each frame is a numbered box that presents a new piece of information or that asks you to respond in some way—sometimes both! When you need to respond, write your response or answer in the space provided. The appropriate response or answer appears in the answer column running along the outside of each page. Just fold over the cover flaps to hide the answers while you read and respond, and lift them up to check your work. Now, let's get used to working with frames.

Working With Frames

1

The heading directly above this frame indicates the beginning of a series of frames that cover a single topic. You don't have to learn an entire chapter all at once. You should, however, finish all the frames between one frame heading and the next before stopping. Remember, _____ headings indicate the beginning of a new topic or concept.

frame

2

You'll learn information in small sections called _____. This is a frame. Most times, you will need to answer a question or complete a statement. To do this, write your response in the _____ provided within the frame.

frames

space

3

Cover the answer columns running along the outside edges of each page using the special cover flaps. Answer each _____ or complete each _____. Immediately check your answer by lifting the flap to uncover the answer column.

question
phrase

4

It is important to check your answer _____ after you have written it down. This will allow you to correct mislearned information.

immediately

5

Move on to the next frame in a chapter only if your answer is correct. Do not be concerned if you make a mistake. Simply go back, find your error, and _____ it. Then move forward, confident you have learned the material.

correct

--- 6 ---

You will practice each learned concept by completing a **Now You Try It** exercise. You will find these exercises at the end of each frame sequence. The **Now You Try It** exercises provide you with an opportunity to test your understanding of the new _____.

concepts

--- 7 ---

If your answer for a **Now You Try It** exercise is wrong, find your mistake and correct it. The answer column shows the steps involved to get the correct answer. If you get more than one wrong, go back and review the preceding frames. It is important to correct _____ _____.

mislearned information

--- 8 ---

Three special, easy-to-read boxes highlight important information in each chapter. **Remember** boxes review concepts, **Did You Notice?** boxes show relationships between concepts, and a **What You've Achieved!** box summarizes the chapter.

--- 9 ---

Each **Remember** box summarizes or reinforces a key concept, procedure, or outcome. You will use this box as a review to check your _____ of previously learned information.

understanding

> REMEMBER
>
> **Check your answer *immediately* after you have written it down. Proceed to the next frame only if your answer is correct.**

--- 10 ---

Each **Did You Notice?** box points out important information not covered in a frame. Use the _____ _____ _____ boxes to expand your knowledge or see the relationship between two concepts.

Did You Notice?

─── **11** ───

Finally, a **What You've Achieved!** box, located at the end of each chapter before the practice test, summarizes basic competencies or concepts you have learned in the chapter. Directions for the review test are included. Use the **What You've Achieved!** box to review the skills you have mastered before working the _____ _____.

review test

─── **12** ───

A review test is placed at the _____ of each chapter. Take the review test to check your understanding of the chapter content.

end

─── **13** ───

Check your answers with the answers found at the end of the review test after you have completed the practice test. Use the _____ _____ _____ box to determine a passing score.

What You've Achieved!

─── **14** ───

Writing your answer down and checking for correctness will _____ the information learned.

reinforce

─── **15** ───

Move on to the next chapter only if you pass each section of the review test. If you do not pass a section in the review test, simply go back and review that section of the chapter and _____ your misunderstanding. Then, and only then, move on to the next chapter, confident you have mastered the necessary competencies.

correct

What You've Achieved!

★ You know how to work with the frame format.

★ You always remember to check your responses immediately.

★ You've learned about the **Remember, Did You Notice?** and **What You've Achieved!** boxes.

Fantastic! What you've learned in this section will help you use this book to learn how to calculate drug dosages accurately. Now, move forward to the math pretest to evaluate your basic number skills.

BASIC NUMBER SKILLS

☆ YOU WILL NEED TO USE BASIC NUMBER skills in order to calculate drug dosages accurately. The four chapters in this section review Roman numerals and Arabic numbers, fractions, decimals, and solving for unknown quantities. To get started, take the math pretest that begins on the next page. If you do well, you may be able to skip to Chapter 5.

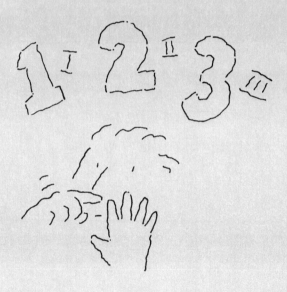

Math Pretest

The pretest is provided to assess your basic math skills and help determine the extent of math review you need to accurately calculate drug dosages. Complete each section below. If more than one answer per section is wrong, review the corresponding content in Chapters 1 through 4. Skip to Chapter 5 only if you get no more than one wrong in **all** sections. Answers are found at the end of the pretest.

Change Roman Numerals to Arabic Numbers

1. XIV = _____

2. VIII = _____

3. XXVII = _____

4. XIX = _____

5. XXXVI = _____

Change Improper Fractions to Mixed Numbers

1. $\dfrac{19}{3}$ = _____

2. $\dfrac{38}{7}$ = _____

3. $\dfrac{18}{4}$ = _____

4. $\dfrac{22}{6}$ = _____

5. $\dfrac{28}{5}$ = _____

Change Mixed Numbers to Improper Fractions

1. $3\dfrac{5}{8}$ = _____

2. $9\dfrac{5}{7}$ = _____

3. $2\dfrac{3}{4}$ = _____

4. $4\dfrac{2}{9}$ = _____

5. $1\frac{13}{14} =$ _____

Add Fractions

1. $\frac{1}{4} + \frac{3}{8} + \frac{1}{3} =$ _____   **2.** $\frac{1}{10} + \frac{3}{5} + 1\frac{3}{4} =$ _____

3. $1\frac{1}{3} + \frac{1}{4} + \frac{1}{6} =$ _____   **4.** $\frac{7}{8} + \frac{1}{2} + \frac{1}{4} =$ _____

5. $\frac{1}{15} + \frac{4}{5} + \frac{2}{3} =$ _____

Subtract Fractions

1. $\frac{8}{9} - \frac{2}{3} =$ _____   **2.** $1\frac{4}{10} - \frac{3}{5} =$ _____

3. $2\frac{1}{4} - \frac{3}{8} =$ _____   **4.** $\frac{12}{15} - \frac{1}{3} =$ _____

5. $\frac{7}{12} - \frac{2}{4} =$ _____

Multiply Fractions

1. $\frac{2}{3} \times \frac{3}{4} =$ _____   **2.** $2\frac{1}{5} \times 15 =$ _____

3. $\frac{9}{12} \times 1\frac{1}{2} =$ _____   **4.** $\frac{8}{9} \times \frac{4}{5} =$ _____

5. $3 \times 1\frac{3}{7} =$ _____

Divide Fractions

1. $\dfrac{2}{3} \div \dfrac{6}{8} =$ _____

2. $1\dfrac{1}{4} \div 2\dfrac{1}{3} =$ _____

3. $\dfrac{9}{10} \div \dfrac{3}{4} =$ _____

4. $1\dfrac{1}{2} \div 2\dfrac{4}{5} =$ _____

5. $\dfrac{11}{12} \div \dfrac{6}{7} =$ _____

Add Decimals

1. $2.01 + 1.1 + 3.003 =$ _____

2. $6.75 + 3.42 + 3.001 =$ _____

3. $2.5 + 0.12 + 0.9 =$ _____

4. $1.033 + 0.67 + 2.508 =$ _____

5. $2.5 + 3.3 + 5.4 =$ _____

Subtract Decimals

1. $23.4 - 4.762 =$ _____

2. $1.099 - 0.177 =$ _____

3. $23.01 - 6.909 =$ _____

4. $5.5 - 2.3 =$ _____

5. $67 - 0.999 =$ _____

Multiply Decimals

1. $15.1 \times 0.34 =$ _____

2. $2.01 \times 82.5 =$ _____

3. $9 \times 1.0278 =$ _____   **4.** $6.75 \times 90.01 =$ _____

5. $20.5 \times 7.25 =$ _____

Divide Decimals

1. $0.75 \div 3 =$ _____   **2.** $2.75 \div 5.5 =$ _____

3. $20.14 \div 0.08 =$ _____   **4.** $0.975 \div 0.025 =$ _____

5. $52.785 \div 0.345 =$ _____

Answers to Pretest

Roman Numerals (review found in Chapter 1)

1. 14   2. 8   3. 27   4. 19   5. 36

Improper Fractions (review found in Chapter 2)

1. $6\frac{1}{3}$ 2. $5\frac{3}{7}$ 3. $4\frac{1}{2}$ 4. $3\frac{2}{3}$ 5. $5\frac{3}{5}$

Mixed Numbers (review found in Chapter 2)

1. $\frac{29}{8}$ 2. $\frac{68}{7}$ 3. $\frac{11}{4}$ 4. $\frac{38}{9}$ 5. $\frac{27}{14}$

Add Fractions (review found in Chapter 2)

1. $\frac{1}{4} = \frac{6}{24}$ 2. $\frac{1}{10} = \frac{2}{20}$ 3. $1\frac{1}{3} = 1\frac{4}{12}$

$\frac{3}{8} = \frac{9}{24}$ $\frac{3}{5} = \frac{12}{20}$ $\frac{1}{4} = \frac{3}{12}$

$\frac{1}{3} = \frac{8}{24}$ $1\frac{3}{4} = 1\frac{15}{20}$ $\frac{1}{6} = \frac{2}{12}$

$\frac{23}{24}$ $1\frac{29}{20} = 2\frac{9}{20}$ $1\frac{9}{12} = 1\frac{3}{4}$

---

4. $\dfrac{7}{8} = \dfrac{7}{8}$

$\quad\ \dfrac{1}{2} = \dfrac{4}{8}$

$\quad\ \dfrac{1}{4} = \dfrac{2}{8}$

$\quad\ \rule{1.5cm}{0.4pt}$

$\qquad\ \dfrac{13}{8} = 1\dfrac{5}{8}$

5. $\dfrac{1}{15} = \dfrac{1}{15}$

$\quad\ \dfrac{4}{5} = \dfrac{12}{15}$

$\quad\ \dfrac{2}{3} = \dfrac{10}{15}$

$\quad\ \rule{1.5cm}{0.4pt}$

$\qquad\ \dfrac{23}{15} = 1\dfrac{8}{15}$

Subtract Fractions (review found in Chapter 2)

1. $\dfrac{8}{9} = \dfrac{8}{9}$

$\quad\ \dfrac{2}{3} = \dfrac{6}{9}$

$\quad\ \rule{1.5cm}{0.4pt}$

$\qquad\ \dfrac{2}{9}$

2. $1\dfrac{4}{10} = \dfrac{14}{10}$

$\quad\ \dfrac{3}{5} = \dfrac{6}{10}$

$\quad\ \rule{1.5cm}{0.4pt}$

$\qquad\ \dfrac{8}{10} = \dfrac{4}{5}$

3. $2\dfrac{1}{4} = 1\dfrac{10}{8}$

$\quad\ \dfrac{3}{8} = \dfrac{3}{8}$

$\quad\ \rule{1.5cm}{0.4pt}$

$\qquad\ 1\dfrac{7}{8}$

---

4. $\dfrac{12}{15} = \dfrac{12}{15}$

$\quad\ \dfrac{1}{3} = \dfrac{5}{15}$

$\quad\ \rule{1.5cm}{0.4pt}$

$\qquad\ \dfrac{7}{15}$

5. $\dfrac{7}{12} = \dfrac{7}{12}$

$\quad\ \dfrac{2}{4} = \dfrac{6}{12}$

$\quad\ \rule{1.5cm}{0.4pt}$

$\qquad\ \dfrac{1}{12}$

Multiply Fractions (review found in Chapter 2)

1. $\dfrac{2}{3} \times \dfrac{3}{4} = \dfrac{6}{12} = \dfrac{1}{2}$

2. $\dfrac{11}{5} \times \dfrac{15}{1} = \dfrac{165}{5} = 33$

---

3. $\dfrac{9}{12} \times \dfrac{3}{2} = \dfrac{27}{24} = 1\dfrac{3}{24} = 1\dfrac{1}{8}$

4. $\dfrac{8}{9} \times \dfrac{4}{5} = \dfrac{32}{45}$

---

5. $\dfrac{3}{1} \times \dfrac{10}{7} = \dfrac{30}{7} = 4\dfrac{2}{7}$

Divide Fractions (review found in Chapter 2)

1. $\dfrac{2}{3} \times \dfrac{8}{6} = \dfrac{16}{18} = \dfrac{8}{9}$

2. $\dfrac{5}{4} \times \dfrac{3}{7} = \dfrac{15}{28}$

---

3. $\dfrac{9}{10} \times \dfrac{4}{3} = \dfrac{36}{30} = 1\dfrac{6}{30} = 1\dfrac{1}{5}$ **4.** $\dfrac{3}{2} \times \dfrac{5}{14} = \dfrac{15}{28}$

5. $\dfrac{11}{12} \times \dfrac{7}{6} = \dfrac{77}{72} = 1\dfrac{5}{72}$

Add Decimals (review found in Chapter 3)

1.	2.	3.	4.	5.
2.010	6.750	2.50	1.033	2.5
1.100	3.420	0.12	0.670	3.3
3.003	3.001	0.90	2.508	5.4
6.113	13.171	3.52	4.211	11.2

Subtract Decimals (review found in Chapter 3)

1.	2.	3.	4.	5.
23.400	1.099	23.010	5.5	67.000
4.762	0.177	6.909	2.3	0.999
18.638	0.922	16.101	3.2	66.001

Multiply Decimals (review found in Chapter 3)

1.	2.	3.
15.1	82.5	1.0278
0.34	2.01	9
604	825	9.2502
453	16500	
5.134	165.825	

4.	5.
90.01	20.5
6.75	7.25
45005	1025
63007	410
54006	1435
607.5675	148.625

Divide Decimals (review found in Chapter 3)

1.
$$3\overline{)0.75} \quad \begin{array}{r} 0.25 \\ \hline 6 \\ \hline 15 \end{array}$$

2.
$$5.5\overline{)2.75} \quad \begin{array}{r} 0.5 \\ \hline 275 \end{array}$$

3.

```
        2 51.75
.08) 20.14 00
     1 6
     4 1
     4 0
       14
        8
        6 0
        5 6
          40
```

4.

```
          39.
.025) .975
       75
      225
      225
```

5.

```
          153.
.345) 52.785
      34 5
      18 28
      17 25
       1 035
       1 035
```

Number Systems

Objectives

When you finish this chapter, you will be able to:

★ Identify when Arabic numbers and Roman numerals are used in administering medications.

★ Convert Roman numerals to Arabic numbers.

★ Convert Arabic numbers to Roman numerals.

Chapter Outline

★ Using Arabic Numbers and Roman Numerals

★ Writing Roman Numerals

★ Addition Rule for Reading Roman Numerals

★ Subtraction Rule for Reading Roman Numerals

Introduction

Arabic Numbers

Two number systems may be used when administering medications. The **Arabic number system** is most commonly used. Arabic numbers can be written as:

whole numbers: 0, 1, 2, 3, 4, 5, 6, 7, 8, 9

fractions: $\dfrac{1}{2}, \dfrac{3}{16}, \dfrac{33}{100}$

decimals: 0.1, 0.02, 0.003

and ratios: 1:2, 3:6, 2:5

The Arabic number system is used to write medication orders in the metric and household systems of weights and measures. (You will learn about these measures in Chapters 5 and 7, respectively.) You will use Arabic numbers to calculate all drug dosages.

Roman Numerals

Roman numerals are only used to write, not calculate, some drug dosages in the apothecary system of weights and measures. (You will learn about this system in Chapter 6.) Roman numerals used to record apothecary weights and measures represent whole numbers.

A combination of seven basic symbols are used to express the numeric values appearing as Roman numerals. The seven symbols may be uppercase or lowercase in form. Throughout this chapter, uppercase Roman numerals are used for clarity. The Roman numeral symbols and corresponding Arabic values are shown in Table 1.1.

TABLE 1.1 **Roman Numeral Symbols**

Roman Numerals		Arabic Numbers
I or i	=	1
V or v	=	5
X or x	=	10
L or l	=	50
C or c	=	100
D or d	=	500
M or m	=	1,000

In practice, Roman numerals above 30 are seldom used to express dosages in the apothecary system of weights and measures. Therefore, only Roman numerals up to 30 will be considered in this chapter.

Using Arabic Numbers and Roman Numerals

1

The most commonly used number system is the _____ number system.

Arabic

--------------------- **2** ---------------------

Arabic numbers are used to write drug dosages in the _____ and household systems of weights and measures.

metric

--------------------- **3** ---------------------

When calculating drug dosages only _____ numbers are used.

Arabic

--------------------- **4** ---------------------

Roman numerals are used to write drug dosages in the _____ system of weights and measures.

apothecary

Writing Roman Numerals

--------------------- **5** ---------------------

Numeric values are expressed as Roman numerals using a combination of _____ symbols.

seven

--------------------- **6** ---------------------

The seven symbols include I, _____, _____, L, C, D, and M.

V, X

--------------------- **7** ---------------------

When expressing dosages, Roman numerals rarely exceed _____ in value.

30

--------------------- **8** ---------------------

The Roman numeral X is the same as _____ in the Arabic number system.

10

V

1

numeric value

10 + 1 = 11

10 + 5 + 1 = 16

9

The Arabic number 5 is the same as the Roman numeral
_____.

10

The Roman numeral I is the same as the Arabic number
_____.

Addition Rule for Reading Roman Numerals

11

The combination of symbols in a Roman numeral expresses
its _____.

12

Two basic rules apply when interpreting Roman numerals. The
first is the **addition rule**. If the first Roman numeral is equal or
greater in value than the following numerals, add the numerals
to determine the total value. For example,

$$VI = 5 + 1 = 6 \quad or \quad XV = 10 + 5 = 15$$

Let's apply this rule:

The value of XI is _____.

13

The value of XVI is _____.

──────────── **14** ────────────

Likewise, when converting an Arabic number to a Roman numeral, apply the addition rule in reverse. Arrange the Roman numeral symbols left to right, from highest to lowest value. For example,

$$21 = 10 + 10 + 1 = XXI$$

Try this example:

17 is expressed as _____ in Roman numerals.

$10 + 5 + 1 + 1 = XVII$

──────────── **15** ────────────

The Roman numeral for 12 is _____.

$12 = 10 + 1 + 1 = XII$

──────────── **16** ────────────

The symbols I and X can be repeated up to three times in a row in a Roman numeral—never more than that. For example,

$$7 = 5 + 1 + 1 = VII$$

or

$$13 = 10 + 1 + 1 + 1 = XIII$$

Try this one:

The Roman numeral for 8 is _____.

$5 + 1 + 1 + 1 = VIII$

──────────── **17** ────────────

The number 18 is written as _____ in Roman numerals.

$10 + 5 + 1 + 1 + 1 =$ XVIII

DID YOU NOTICE?

Repeating the Roman numerals I or X twice doubles the value, while repeating them three times triples the value.

18

The Roman numeral V (5) is never repeated successively because its value when repeated is equal to the Roman numeral X. For example,

$$10 = X, \text{not VV.}$$

Let's try this:

10 + 10 = XX

The Roman numeral for 20 is _____, not XVV.

19
---

10 + 10 + 1 + 1 + 1 = XXIII

The number 23 is written as _____ in Roman numerals.

Subtraction Rule for Reading Roman Numerals

20

The second rule, the **subtraction rule**, states that when one Roman numeral is less than the numeral following it to the right, the smaller numeral is subtracted from the larger numeral. For example,

$$IX = 10 - 1 = 9$$

or

$$XIV = 10 + (5 - 1) = 14$$

Apply the subtraction rule:

5 − 1 = 4

The value of IV is _____.

21
---

10 + (10 − 1) = 19

The value of XIX is _____.

---------------------- **22** ----------------------

Remember, the symbols I and X cannot occur more than three times. If it seems necessary to repeat I or X more than three times when converting Arabic numbers to Roman numerals, apply the subtraction rule in reverse. Arrange the Roman numerals from left to right, the lower value preceding the higher value. For example,

$$4 = 5 - 1 = IV$$

or

$$19 = 10 + (10 - 1) = XIX$$

DID YOU NOTICE?

Some Roman numerals require both addition and subtraction to determine the value.

---------------------- **23** ----------------------

The number 9 is expressed as _____ in Roman numerals.

$10 - 1 = IX$

---------------------- **24** ----------------------

The Roman numeral for 24 is _____.

$10 + 10 + (5 - 1) =$ XXIV

REMEMBER

The Roman numeral V (5) is never repeated successively because its value when repeated is equal to the Roman numeral X.

⭐ What You've Achieved!

★ You've learned to express Arabic numbers 1 through 30 as Roman numerals.

★ You know how to add the values of Roman numerals if the first numeral is equal or greater in value than the following numerals.

★ You know how to interpret numerical values expressed as Roman numerals.

★ You always remember to subtract the lesser Roman numeral when it precedes a larger Roman numeral.

Fantastic! What you've learned in this chapter will help you express and calculate drug dosages. Before moving forward, take the review test to demonstrate your mastery of number systems. If you get more than two wrong in any section, consider reviewing that portion of the chapter again.

Review Test

A

Answer the following questions.

1. When are Arabic numbers used in administering medications? _____

   _____

2. When are Roman numerals used in administering medications? _____

   _____

B

Convert these Arabic numbers to Roman numerals.

3. 2 = _____   4. 3 = _____   5. 4 = _____

6. 8 = _____   7. 9 = _____   8. 24 = _____

9. 29 = _____   10. 18 = _____   11. 23 = _____

-- **c** --

Convert these Roman numerals to Arabic numbers.

12. XV = _____   13. XII = _____   14. XXI = _____

15. XXX = _____   16. XXV = _____   17. IV = _____

18. XIV = _____   19. XXVIII = _____   20. XVII = _____

Answers for Review Test

1. Writing medication orders in the metric and household systems of weights and measures and calculating all drug dosages.

2. Writing some drug dosages in the apothecary system of weights and measures.

3. 1 + 1 = II   4. 1 + 1 + 1 = III   5. 5 − 1 = IV

6. 5 + 1 + 1 + 1 = VIII   7. 10 − 1 = IX

8. 10 + 10 + (5 − 1) = XXIV   9. 10 + 10 + (10 − 1) = XXIX

10. 10 + 5 + 1 + 1 + 1 = XVIII   11. 10 + 10 + 1 + 1 + 1 = XXIII

12. 10 + 5 = 15   13. 10 + 1 + 1 = 12   14. 10 + 10 + 1 = 21

15. 10 + 10 + 10 = 30   16. 10 + 10 + 5 = 25   17. 5 − 1 = 4

18. 10 + (5 − 1) = 14   19. 10 + 10 + 5 + 1 + 1 + 1 = 28

20. 10 + 5 + 1 + 1 = 17

Fractions

Objectives

When you finish this chapter, you will be able to:

★ Define a proper fraction, an improper fraction, and a mixed number.

★ Reduce fractions to their lowest terms.

★ Add, subtract, multiply, and divide fractions.

Chapter Outline

★ Types of Fractions
★ Reducing Fractions
★ Working with Improper Fractions
★ Working with Mixed Numbers
★ Adding Fractions
★ Subtracting Fractions
★ Multiplying Fractions
★ Dividing Fractions

Introduction

A fraction indicates the division of a whole into a number of equal parts. Examples include $\frac{1}{2}$, $\frac{1}{4}$, and $\frac{2}{3}$. The line separating the top and bottom number is a division sign. The number below the line is called the **denominator**. The number above the line is called the **numerator**. The denominator indicates the total number of parts into which the whole number is divided. The numerator indicates the number of parts that are being considered or used. For example:

$$\frac{2}{3} \quad \begin{array}{l} \leftarrow \text{numerator (2 parts are being considered)} \\ \leftarrow \text{denominator (the whole is divided into 3 equal parts)} \end{array}$$

Types of fractions may include proper fractions, improper fractions, and mixed numbers. A **proper fraction** has a numerator that is smaller in value than the denominator, such as $\frac{2}{5}$ or $\frac{5}{8}$. An **improper fraction** has a numerator that is equal to or greater in value than the denominator, such as $\frac{5}{2}$ or $\frac{8}{3}$. A **mixed number** contains a whole number and a proper fraction, such as $1\frac{2}{3}$ or $2\frac{7}{9}$.

You will use fractions primarily to calculate drug dosages in the apothecary system of weights and measures.

Types of Fractions

1

_____ are used to express a portion of a whole number.

Fractions

2

A proper fraction has a top number, called the _____, that is smaller than the bottom number, called the _____.

numerator
denominator

3

The denominator of a proper fraction is _____ than the numerator.

larger

4

An improper fraction has a denominator that is _____ than the numerator.

smaller

5

A fraction that contains a whole number and a proper fraction is called a _____ _____.

mixed number

> **DID YOU NOTICE?**
>
> A proper fraction's value is less than 1.
> An improper fraction's value is equal to or greater than 1.
> A mixed number's value is greater than 1.

---------- **6** ----------

Now You Try It

Identify which fraction is a proper fraction, an improper fraction, and a mixed number.

a. proper fraction

a. $\dfrac{13}{22}$ _____

b. mixed number

b. $4\dfrac{4}{7}$ _____

c. improper fraction

c. $\dfrac{20}{19}$ _____

Reducing Fractions

---------- **7** ----------

A fraction should be reduced to its **lowest terms** because it is easier to work with simpler fractions. Do this by dividing both the numerator and the denominator by the largest whole number that can be divided evenly into them. For example:

$$\frac{8}{12} = \frac{8 \div 4}{12 \div 4} = \frac{2}{3}$$

4 is the largest number that divides evenly into both 8 and 12. Let's apply this rule:

The fraction $\frac{5}{10}$ can be reduced to _____.

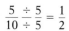

$\dfrac{5 \div 5}{10 \div 5} = \dfrac{1}{2}$

DID YOU NOTICE?

The value of the fraction remains the same as long as you divide the numerator and the denominator by the same number.

---------- **8** ----------

Now You Try It

Express each fraction in its lowest terms.

a. $\dfrac{4}{20} =$ _____

b. $\dfrac{6}{8} =$ _____

c. $\dfrac{24}{72} =$ _____

d. $\dfrac{54}{99} =$ _____

a. $\dfrac{4 \div 4}{20 \div 4} = \dfrac{1}{5}$

b. $\dfrac{6 \div 2}{8 \div 2} = \dfrac{3}{4}$

c. $\dfrac{24 \div 24}{72 \div 24} = \dfrac{1}{3}$

d. $\dfrac{54 \div 9}{99 \div 9} = \dfrac{6}{11}$

Working with Improper Fractions

9

An improper fraction has a numerator that is larger than its denominator. For example, $\frac{3}{2}$ is an improper fraction. To review, the fraction $\frac{7}{9}$ is a _____. $\frac{9}{7}$ is an _____.

proper fraction
improper fraction

10

Change improper fractions to **mixed numbers** to express your answers in the simplest form. Do this by dividing the denominator into the numerator to get the whole number. Place the remainder over the denominator. For example,

$$\dfrac{7}{2} = 2\overline{)7}^{\,3} \longleftarrow \text{whole number}$$
$$\underline{6} $$
$$1 \longleftarrow \text{remainder}$$

$$\dfrac{7}{2} = 3\dfrac{1}{2}$$

Let's try this one. Convert $\frac{21}{6}$ to a mixed number, _____.

$$6\overline{)21}^{\,3} = 3\dfrac{3}{6} = 3\dfrac{1}{2}$$
$$\underline{18}$$
$$3$$

—— **11** ——

Now You Try It

Convert each improper fraction to a mixed number. Reduce the answers to lowest terms.

a. $18\overline{)24}$ $\dfrac{1}{}$ $= 1\dfrac{6}{18} = 1\dfrac{1}{3}$
   $\underline{18}$
   6

a. $\dfrac{24}{18} = $ _____

b. $\dfrac{9}{4} = $ _____

b. $4\overline{)9}$ $\dfrac{2}{}$ $= 2\dfrac{1}{4}$
   $\underline{8}$
   1

c. $\dfrac{13}{3} = $ _____

c. $3\overline{)13}$ $\dfrac{4}{}$ $= 4\dfrac{1}{3}$
   $\underline{12}$
   1

Working with Mixed Numbers

whole number
fraction

—— **12** ——

Mixed numbers, those numbers consisting of a _____ _____ and a _____, can be converted back to improper fractions. Do this when multiplying or dividing a mixed number by another fraction.

—— **13** ——

Convert mixed numbers to improper fractions by multiplying the whole number by the denominator of the fraction. Then add the result to the numerator of the fraction. Place the sum over the denominator. For example,

$$3\dfrac{2}{7} = \dfrac{(3 \times 7)}{7} + \dfrac{2}{7}$$
$$= \dfrac{21}{7} + \dfrac{2}{7}$$
$$= \dfrac{23}{7}$$

$\dfrac{(4 \times 6)}{6} + \dfrac{5}{6} = \dfrac{24}{6} + \dfrac{5}{6}$
$\qquad\qquad = \dfrac{29}{6}$

Apply this rule. Convert $4\dfrac{5}{6}$ to an improper fraction, _____.

Now You Try It

Change each mixed number to an improper fraction.

a. $2\frac{3}{8} =$ _____

b. $3\frac{2}{3} =$ _____

c. $2\frac{3}{5} =$ _____

a. $\frac{(2 \times 8)}{8} + \frac{3}{8} = \frac{19}{8}$

b. $\frac{(3 \times 3)}{3} + \frac{2}{3} = \frac{11}{3}$

c. $\frac{(2 \times 5)}{5} + \frac{3}{5} = \frac{13}{5}$

Adding Fractions

—— 15 ——

You can add fractions if they have a **common denominator**. First, add the numerators. Second, write the sum over the common denominator. For example,

$$\frac{1}{5} + \frac{3}{5} + \frac{4}{5} = \frac{8}{5} = 1\frac{3}{5}$$

Let's try this one. $\frac{2}{9} + \frac{4}{9} =$ _____

Reduce your answer to its lowest terms.

$\frac{6}{9} = \frac{2}{3}$

—— 16 ——

Now You Try It

Add these fractions.

a. $\frac{1}{8} + \frac{3}{8}$ $=$ _____

b. $\frac{2}{7} + \frac{4}{7} + \frac{5}{7}$ $=$ _____

c. $\frac{4}{13} + \frac{5}{13} + \frac{7}{13} + \frac{10}{13} =$ _____

a. $\frac{4}{8} = \frac{1}{2}$

b. $\frac{11}{7} = 1\frac{4}{7}$

c. $\frac{26}{13} = \frac{2}{1} = 2$

To add fractions having different denominators, find the **lowest common denominator**. The lowest common denominator is the smallest whole number that all the denominators in the problem can be evenly divided into. Finding the lowest common denominator is a process of trial and error.

The lowest common denominator is sometimes the largest denominator in a series of fractions. For example, in the series of fractions

$$\frac{1}{2}, \frac{3}{8}, \frac{5}{16}$$

16 is the lowest common denominator because it is the smallest number that 2, 8, and 16 will divide evenly into.

Try this one. The lowest common denominator for $\frac{5}{18}$, $\frac{1}{6}$ and $\frac{2}{3}$ is _____.

18

Two or more of the denominators in a series of fractions may be multiplied together to determine the lowest common denominator. For example, in the series of fractions

$$\frac{1}{10}, \frac{1}{4}, \frac{1}{5}$$

the lowest common denominator is 20 because 20 is the lowest whole number that 10, 4, and 5 will divide evenly into. We get this lowest common denominator by multiplying 4 times 5, then checking to see if the other denominator, 10, will divide evenly into the product, 20. It will, so we have our lowest common denominator. You can see here that finding a lowest common denominator is a process of trial and error. The lowest common denominator for $\frac{2}{7}$ and $\frac{1}{4}$ is _____.

28 (7 × 4)

Now You Try It

Find the lowest common denominator for the following series of fractions.

a. $\dfrac{1}{6}, \dfrac{2}{3}, \dfrac{5}{18}$ _____

b. $\dfrac{7}{36}, \dfrac{5}{6}, \dfrac{2}{9}$ _____

c. $\dfrac{1}{2}, \dfrac{1}{3}, \dfrac{1}{4}$ _____

d. $\dfrac{4}{7}, \dfrac{5}{6}, \dfrac{11}{21}$ _____

a. 18

b. 36

c. 12 (3 × 4)

d. 42 (7 × 6)

20

After finding the lowest common denominator, change each fraction to an **equivalent fraction** containing the lowest common denominator. Do this by multiplying both the numerator and the denominator of the original fraction by the whole number that creates the lowest common denominator. For example, the equivalent fraction of $\frac{2}{7}$ with the lowest common denominator of 28 is $\frac{8}{28}$.

$$\dfrac{2 \times 4 = 8}{7 \times 4 = 28}$$

$$\dfrac{2}{7} = \dfrac{8}{28}$$

The equivalent fraction of $\frac{1}{4}$ with the lowest common denominator of 28 is _____.

$\dfrac{1}{4} \times \dfrac{7}{7} = \dfrac{7}{28}$

 DID YOU NOTICE?

Fractions in which the numerator and denominator have the same value are equal to 1.

21

Finally, add the numerators of each equivalent fraction and place the sum over the common denominator. For example,

$$\dfrac{3}{5} + \dfrac{1}{3} + \dfrac{4}{15} = \dfrac{9}{15} + \dfrac{5}{15} + \dfrac{4}{15}$$

$$= \dfrac{18}{15} = 1\dfrac{3}{15} = 1\dfrac{1}{5}$$

$$\frac{6}{12} + \frac{4}{12} + \frac{3}{12} = \frac{13}{12}$$
$$= 1\frac{1}{12}$$

Solve this problem,

$$\frac{1}{2} + \frac{1}{3} + \frac{1}{4} = \underline{\hspace{3cm}}$$

and reduce the answer to its lowest terms.

---- **22** ----

Now You Try It

Add the following fractions. Reduce the answers to lowest terms.

a. $\frac{13}{14}$

a. $\frac{5}{7} + \frac{3}{14}$ $= \underline{\hspace{2.5cm}}$

b. $\frac{28}{15} = 1\frac{13}{15}$

b. $\frac{2}{3} + \frac{3}{5} + \frac{9}{15} = \underline{\hspace{2.5cm}}$

c. $\frac{31}{24} = 1\frac{7}{24}$

c. $\frac{1}{3} + \frac{1}{4} + \frac{17}{24} = \underline{\hspace{2.5cm}}$

d. $\frac{65}{36} = 1\frac{29}{36}$

d. $\frac{3}{4} + \frac{5}{6} + \frac{2}{9} = \underline{\hspace{2.5cm}}$

 REMEMBER
Reduce all answers to lowest terms.

Subtracting Fractions

---- **23** ----

You subtract fractions by changing them to equivalent fractions with the lowest common denominator. Subtract the numerators, placing the answer over the common denominator. Reduce fractions to lowest terms. For example,

$$\frac{17}{18} - \frac{2}{3} = \frac{17}{18} - \frac{12}{18} = \frac{5}{18}$$

Let's apply this rule:

Solve the problem, $1\frac{1}{7} - \frac{5}{6} = $ _____

$$\frac{8}{7} - \frac{5}{6} = \frac{48}{42} - \frac{35}{42} = \frac{13}{42}$$

REMEMBER

Change mixed fractions to improper fractions before subtracting.

───────── **24** ─────────

Now You Try It

Solve each problem. Reduce the answers to lowest terms.

a. $\frac{11}{12} - \frac{3}{12} = $ _____

b. $\frac{7}{10} - \frac{3}{10} = $ _____

c. $\frac{2}{3} - \frac{1}{9} = $ _____

d. $2\frac{1}{2} - \frac{7}{8} = $ _____

a. $\frac{8}{12} = \frac{2}{3}$

b. $\frac{4}{10} = \frac{2}{5}$

c. $\frac{6}{9} - \frac{1}{9} = \frac{5}{9}$

d. $\frac{5}{2} - \frac{7}{8} = \frac{20}{8} - \frac{7}{8}$

$\quad = \frac{13}{8} = 1\frac{5}{8}$

Multiplying Fractions

───────── **25** ─────────

Multiply fractions by multiplying the numerators and then the denominators. For example,

$$\frac{3}{4} \times \frac{2}{5} = \frac{3 \times 2}{4 \times 5} \longleftarrow \text{numerators multiplied}$$
$$\longleftarrow \text{denominators multiplied}$$
$$= \frac{6}{20} = \frac{3}{10}$$

Let's try a multiplication problem. Reduce the answer to lowest terms.

$$\frac{3 \times 5}{16 \times 6} = \frac{15}{96} = \frac{5}{32}$$

$$\frac{3}{16} \times \frac{5}{6} = \underline{\hspace{2cm}}$$

26

To multiply a whole number by a fraction, first change the whole number to a fraction by placing the whole number over 1.

multiplying the numera-
tors

multiplying the denomi-
nators

The new numerator is obtained by _____ _____. The new denominator is obtained by _____ _____ _____. For example,

$$4 \times \frac{1}{3} = \frac{4 \times 1}{1 \times 3} \longleftarrow \text{numerators multiplied}$$
$$\longleftarrow \text{denominators multiplied}$$

$$= \frac{4}{3} = 1\frac{1}{3}$$

Try this one. Reduce the answer to lowest terms.

$$\frac{3 \times 12}{1 \times 13} = \frac{36}{13} = 2\frac{10}{13}$$

$$3 \times \frac{12}{13} = \underline{\hspace{2cm}}$$

27

Now You Try It

Multiply the following fractions. Reduce answers to lowest terms.

a. $\frac{2 \times 1}{3 \times 2} = \frac{2}{6} = \frac{1}{3}$

a. $\frac{2}{3} \times \frac{1}{2} = \underline{\hspace{1.5cm}}$

b. $\frac{3}{4} \times \frac{2}{1} = \frac{3 \times 2}{4 \times 1} = \frac{6}{4}$
$= 1\frac{1}{2}$

b. $\frac{3}{4} \times 2 = \underline{\hspace{1.5cm}}$

c. $\frac{5 \times 3}{6 \times 20} = \frac{15}{120} = \frac{1}{8}$

c. $\frac{5}{6} \times \frac{3}{20} = \underline{\hspace{1.5cm}}$

d. $6 \times \frac{2}{3} = \frac{6 \times 2}{1 \times 3} = \frac{12}{3}$
$= 4$

d. $6 \times \frac{2}{3} = \underline{\hspace{1.5cm}}$

Dividing Fractions

─────────────── **28** ───────────────

Divide fractions by converting the division problem to a multiplication problem. Do this by inverting the divisor, which is the fraction to the right of the division sign. For example:

$$\frac{1}{5} \div \frac{1}{2}$$

$$\uparrow \qquad \uparrow$$

Dividend   Divisor

$$= \frac{1}{5} \times \frac{2}{1} = \frac{1 \times 2}{5 \times 1} = \frac{2}{5}$$

Try this division exercise. Reduce the answer to its lowest terms.

$$\frac{6}{7} \div \frac{5}{6} = \underline{\hspace{3cm}}$$

$$\frac{6}{7} \times \frac{6}{5} = \frac{6 \times 6}{7 \times 5} = \frac{36}{35}$$
$$= 1\frac{1}{35}$$

─────────────── **29** ───────────────

To divide a fraction by a whole number, first change the whole number to a fraction. Then, invert the divisor and multiply. For example,

$$\frac{4}{5} \div 2 = \frac{4}{5} \div \frac{2}{1} = \frac{4}{5} \times \frac{1}{2} = \frac{4}{10} = \frac{2}{5}$$

Solve this problem, and reduce the answer to its lowest terms.

$$5 \div \frac{7}{8} = \underline{\hspace{3cm}}$$

$$\frac{5}{1} \div \frac{7}{8} = \frac{5}{1} \times \frac{8}{7} = \frac{40}{7}$$
$$= 5\frac{5}{7}$$

─────────────── **30** ───────────────

Now You Try It

Divide the following fractions. Reduce the answers to lowest terms.

a. $\dfrac{7}{8} \times \dfrac{4}{1} = \dfrac{7 \times 4}{8 \times 1} = \dfrac{28}{8}$

$\qquad = 3\dfrac{4}{8} = 3\dfrac{1}{2}$

b. $\dfrac{1}{3} \times \dfrac{12}{7} = \dfrac{1 \times 12}{3 \times 7}$

$\qquad = \dfrac{12}{21} = \dfrac{4}{7}$

c. $\dfrac{3}{4} \times \dfrac{4}{3} = \dfrac{3 \times 4}{4 \times 3}$

$\qquad = \dfrac{12}{12} = 1$

a. $\dfrac{7}{8} \div \dfrac{1}{4} =$ _____

b. $\dfrac{1}{3} \div \dfrac{7}{12} =$ _____

c. $\dfrac{3}{4} \div \dfrac{3}{4} =$ _____

☆ What You've Achieved!

★ You've learned to distinguish between proper and improper fractions.

★ You always remember to reduce fractions to their lowest terms.

★ You know how to add, subtract, multiply, and divide fractions.

Great work! What you've learned in this chapter will help you in calculating dosages in the apothecary system of weights and measures. Before moving forward, take the review test to demonstrate your mastery of fractions. If you get more than one question wrong in any section, consider studying that portion of the chapter again.

Review Test: Reduce All Answers to Lowest Terms

A

Reduce the following fractions to lowest terms.

1. $\dfrac{9}{36} =$ _____

2. $\dfrac{45}{90} =$ _____

Change the improper fractions to mixed numbers.

3. $\dfrac{86}{25} =$ _____   4. $\dfrac{19}{3} =$ _____

Change the mixed numbers to improper fractions.

5. $3\dfrac{1}{10} =$ _____   6. $2\dfrac{5}{8} =$ _____

Add the following fractions.

7. $\dfrac{1}{3} + \dfrac{1}{4} + \dfrac{1}{6} =$ _____   8. $\dfrac{2}{4} + \dfrac{1}{4} =$ _____   9. $\dfrac{1}{2} + \dfrac{1}{3} + \dfrac{1}{5} =$ _____

Subtract the following fractions.

10. $\dfrac{5}{7} - \dfrac{2}{7} =$ _____   11. $\dfrac{6}{7} - \dfrac{2}{3} =$ _____   12. $1\dfrac{2}{3} - \dfrac{7}{9} =$ _____

Multiply the following fractions.

13. $\dfrac{5}{12} \times \dfrac{4}{9} =$ _____   14. $\dfrac{4}{5} \times \dfrac{5}{7} =$ _____   15. $2 \times \dfrac{3}{5} =$ _____

16. $\dfrac{4}{7} \times 3 =$ _____

Divide the following fractions.

17. $\dfrac{1}{5} \div \dfrac{3}{20} =$ _____   18. $\dfrac{2}{7} \div \dfrac{3}{4} =$ _____   19. $\dfrac{6}{7} \div \dfrac{3}{5} =$ _____

20. $\dfrac{1}{3} \div 5 =$ _____

Answers for Review Test

1. $\dfrac{9 \div 9}{36 \div 9} = \dfrac{1}{4}$

2. $\dfrac{45 \div 45}{90 \div 45} = \dfrac{1}{2}$

3. $25\overline{)86} \;\begin{array}{c}3\\ \end{array}= 3\dfrac{11}{25}$ $\dfrac{75}{11}$

---

4. $3\overline{)19}\;\begin{array}{c}6\\ \end{array} = 6\dfrac{1}{3}$ $\dfrac{18}{1}$

5. $\dfrac{(3 \times 10)}{10} + \dfrac{1}{10} = \dfrac{31}{10}$

6. $\dfrac{(2 \times 8)}{8} + \dfrac{5}{8} = \dfrac{21}{8}$

7. $\dfrac{1}{3} + \dfrac{1}{4} + \dfrac{1}{6} = \dfrac{4}{12} + \dfrac{3}{12} + \dfrac{2}{12} = \dfrac{9}{12} = \dfrac{3}{4}$

8. $\dfrac{2}{4} + \dfrac{1}{4} = \dfrac{3}{4}$

---

9. $\dfrac{1}{2} + \dfrac{1}{3} + \dfrac{1}{5} = \dfrac{15}{30} + \dfrac{10}{30} + \dfrac{6}{30} = \dfrac{31}{30} + 1\dfrac{1}{30}$

10. $\dfrac{5}{7} - \dfrac{2}{7} = \dfrac{3}{7}$

---

11. $\dfrac{6}{7} - \dfrac{2}{3} = \dfrac{18}{21} - \dfrac{14}{21} = \dfrac{4}{21}$

12. $1\dfrac{2}{3} - \dfrac{7}{9} = \dfrac{5}{3} - \dfrac{7}{9} = \dfrac{15}{9} - \dfrac{7}{9} + \dfrac{8}{9}$

---

13. $\dfrac{5 \times 4}{12 \times 9} = \dfrac{20}{108} = \dfrac{5}{27}$

14. $\dfrac{4 \times 5}{5 \times 7} = \dfrac{20}{35} = \dfrac{4}{7}$

15. $\dfrac{2 \times 3}{1 \times 5} = \dfrac{6}{5} = 1\dfrac{1}{5}$

---

16. $\dfrac{4 \times 3}{7 \times 1} = \dfrac{12}{7} = 1\dfrac{5}{7}$

17. $\dfrac{1 \times 20}{5 \times 3} = \dfrac{20}{15} = \dfrac{4}{3} = 1\dfrac{1}{3}$

18. $\dfrac{2 \times 4}{7 \times 3} = \dfrac{8}{21}$

---

19. $\dfrac{6 \times 5}{7 \times 3} = \dfrac{30}{21} = \dfrac{10}{7} = 1\dfrac{3}{7}$

20. $\dfrac{1 \times 1}{3 \times 5} = \dfrac{1}{15}$

Decimals

Objectives

When you finish this chapter, you will be able to:

★ Define a decimal.
★ Round decimals to the nearest tenth, hundredth, and whole number.
★ Add, subtract, multiply and divide decimals.
★ Convert fractions to decimals.

Chapter Outline

★ Decimal Position and Relative Value
★ Rounding Off Decimals
★ Adding Decimals
★ Subtracting Decimals
★ Multiplying Decimals
★ Dividing Decimals
★ Converting Fractions to Decimals

Introduction

Decimals (decimal fractions) are another way to express parts of a whole number. Decimal numbers are arranged around a **decimal point**. Numbers to the left of the decimal point are whole number powers of ten. Numbers to the right of the decimal point are fractional powers of ten. Decimal names and positions are shown in Table 3.1.

TABLE 3.1 **Decimal Names and Positions**

Whole Numbers	1000.0	= one thousand
	100.0	= one hundred
	10.0	= ten
	1.0	= one
	0.1	= one tenth
	0.01	= one hundredth
Fractions	0.001	= one thousandth

A zero is added to the left of the decimal point when writing a decimal without a whole number, such as 0.125, to emphasize the decimal point and avoid errors. Zeros added to the right of the last number of a decimal do not change its value. For example, the number six written as a decimal is 6.0 and pronounced, "six point zero." Zeros are also used as place holders to put a number in the correct position in relation to the decimal point. For example, 0.05 is five-hundredths.

You will use decimals to calculate and express drug dosages in the metric system of weights and measures.

Decimal Position and Relative Value

1

Decimals

_____ express parts of a whole number.

2

tenth

The first number to the right of the decimal point is in the _____ position.

3

hundredth

The second number to the right of the decimal point is in the _____ position.

4

thousandth

The third number to the right of the decimal point is in the _____ position.

5

The value of a number is indicated by its position relative to the decimal point. The larger the whole number to the left of the decimal point, the greater the value. For example, 6.25 is greater than 1.25.

Try this example: Which number has the higher value, 201.3 or 125.9? _____

201.3

6

If the whole numbers are the same or the whole number is absent, then the decimal with the highest number representing tenths has the greatest value. For example, 0.5 has a greater value than 0.45.

Let's try this one: Which decimal has the higher value, 0.3 or 0.125? _____

0.3

REMEMBER

To avoid errors, zeros are added to the left of the decimal point when writing decimals without whole numbers.

7

The hundredth position is used to determine the value of decimals if the decimals are identical through the tenth position. For example, 0.05 is greater than 0.025. Which decimal has the higher value, 1.125 or 1.11? _____

1.125

In performing dosage calculation, you will not usually be concerned with values less than 0.001.

8

Now You Try It
Choose the decimal with the highest value.

a. 5.245 or 5.056 or 3.99

a. 5.245

b. 0.57 or 0.256 or 0.75

b. 0.75

c. 1.03 or 1.025 or 1.0291

c. 1.03

DID YOU NOTICE?

The number of digits to the right of the decimal point does not indicate the value of the decimal.

Rounding Off Decimals

—————————— **9** ——————————

When calculating dosages in the metric system, the results may need to be rounded off to the nearest whole number, the nearest tenth, or the nearest hundredth, depending on the drug preparation used. When the number to the right of the position to be rounded is **greater than** or **equal to five** (≥ 5), round up by one number, then drop the remaining numbers to the right. For example, let's round 0.16 to the nearest tenth.

0.16   ⟵ (value ≥ 5)

↑

tenths

Therefore:

0.2

Let's apply this rule. Round these decimals to the nearest tenth:

5.78 ⟶ _____

7.16 ⟶ _____

5.8

7.2

—————————— **10** ——————————

When the number to the right of the position to be rounded is **less than five** (< 5), do not change the number to be rounded off. Simply delete the numbers to the right. For example, let's round 0.534 to the nearest hundredth.

0.534   ⟵ (value < 5)

↑

hundredth

Therefore:

0.53

Now let's try rounding these decimals to the nearest hundredth:

1.213 ⟶ _____

8.572 ⟶ _____

1.21

8.57

11

To become more familiar with these rules, consider 2.654. Let's round it to the nearest:

> whole number: 3   (because 6 > 5)
>
> tenth: 2.7   (because 5 = 5)
>
> hundredth: 2.65 (because 4 < 5).

12

Now You Try It

Round the following numbers to the nearest:

	Whole number	Tenth	Hundredth
a. 3.568	_____	_____	_____
b. 4.314	_____	_____	_____

a. 4   3.6   3.57

b. 4   4.3   4.31

REMEMBER

Round up by one number when the number immediately to its right is equal to five.

Adding Decimals

13

To add decimals, place the numbers in a column, keeping the decimal points directly under each other. Then add and carry as necessary. For example:

$$1.2 + 3.75 + 4.0 = \underline{\ ?\ }$$

$$\downarrow$$

$$
\begin{array}{r}
1.2 \\
3.75 \\
+4.0 \\
\hline
8.95 \\
\end{array}
$$

$$\uparrow$$

14

When adding columns of decimals, you may find it helpful to add zeros to the right of the last digit of each number. This will help you align the columns of numbers. For example:

$$0.9 + 3.02 + 12.012 = \underline{\quad ? \quad}$$

$$
\begin{array}{r}
0.900 \\
3.020 \\
+12.012 \\
\end{array}
$$

15.932

15

Now You Try It

Add the following decimals.

a. $432 + 0.02$ $\quad = \underline{\hspace{2cm}}$

b. $2.36 + 5.576$ $\quad = \underline{\hspace{2cm}}$

c. $12.12 + 3.001$ $\quad = \underline{\hspace{2cm}}$

d. $0.005 + 1.05 + 1.5 = \underline{\hspace{2cm}}$

a.
$$
\begin{array}{r}
432.00 \\
+ \quad 0.02 \\
\hline
432.02 \\
\end{array}
$$

b.
$$
\begin{array}{r}
2.360 \\
+5.576 \\
\hline
7.936 \\
\end{array}
$$

c.
$$
\begin{array}{r}
12.120 \\
+ \quad 3.001 \\
\hline
15.121 \\
\end{array}
$$

d.
$$
\begin{array}{r}
0.005 \\
1.050 \\
+1.500 \\
\hline
2.555 \\
\end{array}
$$

Subtracting Decimals

16

When subtracting decimals, place the numbers in a column, keeping the decimal points directly under each other. Add zeros so each number involved in the operation has the same number of digits and the columns align. Then subtract and borrow as necessary. For example:

$$9.54 - 0.621 = \underline{\quad ? \quad}$$
$$\downarrow$$

$$
\begin{array}{r}
9.540 \\
-0.621 \\
\hline
8.919 \\
\end{array}
$$
$$\uparrow$$

Let's apply this rule. Subtract these decimals:

$$3.64 - 1.8 = \underline{\hspace{2cm}}$$

$$\begin{array}{r} 3.64 \\ -1.80 \\ \hline 1.84 \end{array}$$

———————— **17** ————————

Now You Try It

Subtract the following decimals.

a. $4.5 - 1.3 \quad = \underline{\hspace{2cm}}$

b. $1.2 - 0.8 \quad = \underline{\hspace{2cm}}$

c. $85.7 - 4.92 \quad = \underline{\hspace{2cm}}$

d. $0.125 - 0.015 = \underline{\hspace{2cm}}$

a. $\begin{array}{r} 4.5 \\ -1.3 \\ \hline 3.2 \end{array}$ b. $\begin{array}{r} 1.2 \\ -0.8 \\ \hline 0.4 \end{array}$

c. $\begin{array}{r} 85.70 \\ -\ 4.92 \\ \hline 80.78 \end{array}$ d. $\begin{array}{r} 0.125 \\ -0.015 \\ \hline 0.110 \end{array}$

Multiplying Decimals

———————— **18** ————————

Multiplication is an easy two-step process! First, disregard the decimal points and multiply the **multiplicand** (top number) by the **multiplier** (bottom number).

Second, figure the number of decimal places in the **product** (the answer) by counting the total number of decimal spaces in the multiplier and multiplicand. Locate the decimal point the same number of spaces to the left in the product. Add zeros as necessary. For example:

$$2.03 \times 0.024 = \underline{\ ?\ }$$

$$\begin{array}{r} 2.03 \quad \longleftarrow \text{multiplicand} \\ \times 0.0\,24 \quad \longleftarrow \text{multiplier} \\ \hline 8\ 12 \quad\quad\quad\quad\quad \\ 4\ 0\ 6 \quad\quad\quad\quad\quad \\ \hline 4\ 8\ 72 \quad \longleftarrow \text{product} \end{array}$$

There are a total of five decimal spaces in the multiplicand and multiplier, so

$$\begin{array}{c} 0\,4\,8\,7\,2\,. \\ 5\ 4\ 3\ 2\ 1 \end{array}$$

$$
\begin{array}{r}
3.7 \\
\times 0.81 \\
\hline
37 \\
296 \;\;\;\\
\hline
2997
\end{array} = 2.997
$$

0.04872

Let's try a multiplication problem. Multiply these decimals:

$$3.7 \times 0.81 = \underline{\hspace{1.5cm}}$$

--------------------- **19** ---------------------

a.
$$
\begin{array}{r}
2.3\,5 \\
\times 5.1 \\
\hline
2\,3\,5 \\
11\,7\,5\;\;\\
\hline
11\,9\,8\,5
\end{array} = 11.985
$$

b.
$$
\begin{array}{r}
0.8 \\
\times 0.2\,1 \\
\hline
8 \\
1\,6\;\;\\
\hline
1\,6\,8
\end{array} = 0.168
$$

c.
$$
\begin{array}{r}
2.2 \\
\times 4.6 \\
\hline
13\,2 \\
88\;\;\\
\hline
101\,2
\end{array} = 10.12
$$

d.
$$
\begin{array}{r}
1.2 \\
\times 0.3 \\
\hline
3\,6
\end{array} = 0.36
$$

Now You Try It

Multiply the following decimals.

a. $2.35 \times 5.1 = \underline{\hspace{1.5cm}}$

b. $0.8 \times 0.21 = \underline{\hspace{1.5cm}}$

c. $2.2 \times 4.6 \;\; = \underline{\hspace{1.5cm}}$

d. $1.2 \times 0.3 \;\; = \underline{\hspace{1.5cm}}$

Dividing Decimals

--------------------- **20** ---------------------

Division requires a three-step process. First, convert the divisor (the number that does the dividing) to a whole number by moving the decimal point to the right. For example:

$$1.5 \div 0.25 = \underline{\;\;?\;\;}$$

Divisor $\longrightarrow$ $0.25\,\overline{)1.5}$

$$0.\underset{\smile}{2}\,\underset{\smile}{5}.\,\overline{)1.5}$$
$$1\;2$$

Second, move the decimal point in the dividend (the number being divided) the same number of spaces to the right. Add zeros as necessary.

$$25\overline{)1.5\underset{\smile}{}.} \longleftarrow \text{Dividend}$$
$$1\;2$$

$$25\overline{)150.}$$

Third, place the decimal point in the dividend directly above the same space in the quotient (answer) and divide.

Section I BASIC NUMBER SKILLS

$$25\overline{)150.}^{\,\cdot} \quad \longleftarrow \text{Quotient}$$

$$
\begin{array}{r}
6. \\
25\overline{)150.} \\
\underline{150} \\
0
\end{array}
= 6.0
$$

Let's try a division exercise. Solve this problem:

$$0.156 \div 0.06 = \underline{\hspace{2cm}}$$

$$
\begin{array}{r}
2\,.6 \\
0.\underset{\smile}{0}\,\underset{\smile}{6}.\overline{)0.1\underset{\smile}{5}.6} \\
\underline{1\ 2} \\
3\ 6 \\
\underline{3\ 6} \\
0
\end{array}
= 2.6
$$

21

Now You Try It

Divide the following decimals.

a. $0.292 \div 0.4 = \underline{\hspace{2cm}}$

b. $2.134 \div 2.2 = \underline{\hspace{2cm}}$

c. $19.95 \div 2.1 = \underline{\hspace{2cm}}$

d. $0.06 \div 0.5 \ = \underline{\hspace{2cm}}$

a.
$$
\begin{array}{r}
.73 \\
0.4\overline{)\,.2\ 92} \\
\underline{2\ 8} \\
12 \\
\underline{12}
\end{array}
= 0.73
$$

b.
$$
\begin{array}{r}
.97 \\
2.2\overline{)2.1\ 34} \\
\underline{1\ 9\ 8} \\
1\ 5\ 4 \\
\underline{1\ 5\ 4}
\end{array}
= 0.97
$$

Converting Fractions to Decimals

c.
$$
\begin{array}{r}
9.5 \\
2.1\overline{)19.9\ 5} \\
\underline{18\ 9} \\
1\ 0\ 5 \\
\underline{1\ 0\ 5}
\end{array}
= 9.5
$$

22

When calculating liquid medication dosages, it may be necessary to change a fraction into a decimal number. To accomplish this, divide the denominator of the fraction into the numerator. For example:

d.
$$
\begin{array}{r}
.12 \\
0.5\overline{)\,.0\ 60} \\
\underline{5} \\
10 \\
\underline{10}
\end{array}
= 0.12
$$

$$\frac{5}{8} = \underline{\quad ? \quad}$$

$$
\begin{array}{r}
.625 \\
8\overline{)5.000} \\
\underline{4\ 8} \\
20 \\
\underline{16} \\
40
\end{array}
= 0.625
$$

Try this one. Convert the fraction $\frac{3}{16}$ to a decimal number _____.

```
    .1875
16)3.000
    16
   ───
    140
    128
   ───
    120
    112
   ───
     80
```

REMEMBER

Zeros can be added to the right of the last digit in a decimal without changing the numerical value.

─────────── **23** ───────────

Now You Try It

Convert the following fractions to decimals. Round the answers to the nearest hundredth.

a. $\frac{2}{7}$ = _____

b. $\frac{3}{8}$ = _____

c. $\frac{1}{6}$ = _____

d. $\frac{7}{12}$ = _____

REMEMBER

The answer to a division problem must be solved to the thousandths place to round to the nearest hundredth.

a.
```
    .285  = 0.29
 7)2.000
    1 4
   ───
     60
     56
    ───
     40
     35
```

b.
```
    .375  = 0.38
 8)3.000
    2 4
   ───
     60
     56
    ───
     40
     40
```

c.
```
    .165  = 0.17
 6)1.000
     6
    ───
     40
     36
    ───
     40
     30
```

d.
```
    .583  = 0.58
12)7.000
    6 0
   ───
    1 00
      96
    ───
      40
```

⭐ What You've Achieved!

★ You've learned to compare the relative value of two or more decimals.

★ You know how to round decimal numbers.

★ You know how to add, subtract, multiply, and divide decimal numbers.

★ You can convert fractions into decimal numbers.

Great job! What you've learned in this chapter will help you in calculating dosages in the metric and the household systems of weights and measures. Before moving forward, take the review test to demonstrate your mastery of decimals. If you get more than one question wrong in any section, consider reviewing that portion of the chapter.

Review Test

─────────────── **A** ───────────────

Round off the following numbers to the nearest:

		Whole number	Tenth	Hundredth
1.	17.786 =	_____	_____	_____
2.	4.394 =	_____	_____	_____

─────────────── **B** ───────────────

Add the following:

3. 4.6 + 8.01 + 16 = _____   **4.** 0.023 + 1.01 + 3.3 = _____

5. 7.517 + 3.2 + 0.16 = _____

---------- **C** ----------

Subtract the following:

6. $4.7 - 1.824 =$ _____   7. $7.62 - 4.8 =$ _____

8. $0.58 - 0.061 =$ _____

---------- **D** ----------

Multiply the following decimals:

9. $1.2 \times 0.3 =$ _____   10. $21.4 \times 1.2 =$ _____

11. $61.1 \times 0.5 =$ _____   12. $0.25 \times 11.4 =$ _____

---------- **E** ----------

Divide the following decimals and round the answers to the nearest hundredth:

13. $2 \div 0.002 =$ _____   14. $200 \div 2.5 =$ _____

15. $2.513 \div 1.1 =$ _____   16. $0.444 \div 2.12 =$ _____

---------- **F** ----------

Convert the following fractions to decimals. Round the answer to the nearest tenth.

17. $\dfrac{5}{9} =$ _____   18. $\dfrac{3}{5} =$ _____   19. $\dfrac{7}{11} =$ _____

20. $\dfrac{11}{15} =$ _____

Answers for Review Test

1. 18, 17.8, 17.79   2. 4, 4.4, 4.39   3.
$$
\begin{array}{r}
4.60 \\
8.01 \\
+16.00 \\
\hline
28.61
\end{array}
$$

4.
$$
\begin{array}{r}
0.023 \\
1.010 \\
+3.300 \\
\hline
4.333
\end{array}
$$
5.
$$
\begin{array}{r}
7.517 \\
3.200 \\
+0.160 \\
\hline
10.877
\end{array}
$$
6.
$$
\begin{array}{r}
4.700 \\
-1.824 \\
\hline
2.876
\end{array}
$$

7.
$$\begin{array}{r} 7.62 \\ -4.80 \\ \hline 2.82 \end{array}$$

8.
$$\begin{array}{r} 0.580 \\ -0.061 \\ \hline 0.519 \end{array}$$

9.
$$\begin{array}{r} 1.2 \\ \times\, 0.3 \\ \hline 3\ 6 \end{array} = 0.36$$

10.
$$\begin{array}{r} 21.4 \\ \times 1.2 \\ \hline 42\ 8 \\ 214\quad \\ \hline 256\ 8 \end{array} = 25.68$$

11.
$$\begin{array}{r} 61.1 \\ \times 0.5 \\ \hline 305\ 5 \end{array} = 30.55$$

12.
$$\begin{array}{r} 11.4 \\ \times 0.25 \\ \hline 570 \\ 228\quad \\ \hline 2850 \end{array} = 2.850 = 2.85$$

13.
$$0.\underset{\smile}{0}\,\underset{\smile}{0}\,2\,\overline{)2.\underset{\smile}{0}\,\underset{\smile}{0}\,\underset{\smile}{0}\,0.} = 1000$$
quotient $1\ 0\ 0\ 0.$
$\underline{2}$

14.
$$2.\underset{\smile}{5}\,\overline{)200.\underset{\smile}{0}\,.} = 80$$
quotient $8\ 0.$
$\underline{200}$

15.
$$1.\underset{\smile}{1}\,\overline{)2.\underset{\smile}{5}\,.13} = 2.28$$
quotient 2.28
$\underline{2\ 2}$
$\ \ 3\ 1$
$\ \ \underline{2\ 2}$
$\ \ \ \ 93$
$\ \ \ \ \underline{88}$
$\ \ \ \ \ 5$

16.
$$2.\underset{\smile}{1}\,\underset{\smile}{2}\,\overline{).4\,4\,.400} = 0.21$$
quotient $.209$
$\underline{4\ 2\ 4}$
$\ \ 2\ 000$
$\ \ \underline{1\ 908}$

17.
$$9\,\overline{)5.00} = 0.6$$
quotient $.55$
$\underline{4\ 5}$
$\ \ 50$
$\ \ \underline{45}$

18.
$$5\,\overline{)3.00} = 0.6$$
quotient $.60$
$\underline{3\ 0}$

19.
$$11\,\overline{)7.00} = 0.6$$
quotient $.63$
$\underline{6\ 6}$
$\ \ 40$
$\ \ \underline{33}$

20.
$$15\,\overline{)11.00} = .7$$
quotient $.73$
$\underline{10\ 5}$
$\ \ 50$
$\ \ \underline{45}$
$\ \ \ 5$

4

Calculating an Unknown Quantity

Objectives

When you finish this chapter, you will be able to:

★ Define a ratio.

★ Define a proportion.

★ Identify the means and extremes in a proportion.

★ Calculate the value of an unknown quantity using the ratio-and-proportion method.

Chapter Outline

★ Ratios and Proportions

★ Means and Extremes

★ Using Ratios and Proportions to Solve for Unknowns

★ Working with Proportions Containing Fractions

Introduction

Correct calculation of dosages is critical for the safe and accurate administration of medications. Calculating dosages involves determining an unknown quantity. In arithmetic terms, an unknown quantity is represented by x.

The **ratio-and-proportion method** can be used to calculate dosages. This method is the most commonly used method for solving all kinds of dosage calculation problems. It is the safest method because it allows you to easily check your calculations for accuracy.

The ratio-and-proportion method utilizes the previously learned skills of multiplying and dividing whole numbers, fractions, and decimals. You will use the ratio-and-proportion method to calculate dosages throughout the rest of this book.

Ratios and Proportions

—— **1** ——

When calculating dosages, a simple equation can be used to solve for an unknown quantity. This unknown quantity can be represented by ——————.

x

—— **2** ——

A **ratio** is a comparison of two numbers. The two numbers being compared are separated by a colon (:) and the expression is read "is to." The ratio 2 "is to" 5 is written 2:5.

Try this example: The ratio 7 "is to" 10 is written ——————.

7:10

—— **3** ——

A **proportion** is a statement indicating that two ratios are equal. The ratios are separated by an equal (=) sign. For example, 2:5 has the same value as the ratio 6:15. Therefore both ratios can be expressed by the proportion statement 2:5 = 6:15.

Now try this: Express the ratios 8:16 and 1:2 as a proportion. ——————

8:16 = 1:2

Means and Extremes

—— **4** ——

The outside numbers of a proportion are called the **extremes**. For example:

extremes

2:5 = 6:15

The inside numbers are called the **means**. For example:

means

2:5 = 6:15

7 and 30
10 and 21

In the proportion, 7:10 = 21:30, the extremes are _____ and the means are _____.

———————————— **5** ————————————

When you multiply the means together and the extremes together in a proportion, the products are equal. Again using the proportion 2:5 = 6:15 as an example:

$$2 \times 15 = 30 \longleftarrow \text{product of extremes}$$
$$5 \times 6 = 30 \longleftarrow \text{product of means}$$
$$30 = 30$$

This principle verifies that the two ratios are equal and that the statement is indeed a proportion.

Let's apply this rule. Prove the two ratios are equal and the statement 7:10 = 21:30 is a proportion. _____

$7 \times 30 = 210$
$10 \times 21 = 210$
$210 = 210$

———————————— **6** ————————————

Now You Try It

Find the product of the means and the extremes for the following proportions. Determine if each expression is a true proportion.

a. 1:2 = 3:6
  Means = 6
  Extremes = 6
  True proportion

b. 12:9 = 4:3
  Means = 36
  Extremes = 36
  True proportion

c. 8:18 = 2:5
  Means = 36
  Extremes = 40
  Not a true proportion
  as means ≠ extremes

a. 1:2 = 3:6   Means = _____   Extremes = _____

b. 12:9 = 4:3   Means = _____   Extremes = _____

c. 8:18 = 2:5   Means = _____   Extremes = _____

Using Ratios and Proportions to Solve for Unknowns

———————————— **7** ————————————

extremes

The principle that the product of the means is equal to the product of the _____ has its most important application when one of the numbers is unknown.

8

When using ratios and proportions to solve for unknowns, first multiply the means and the extremes. The product containing the unknown (x) should be placed on the left side of the equation to avoid confusion. For example:

means

$$2{:}5 = 6{:}x$$

extremes

$$2 \times (x) = 5 \times 6 \quad \leftarrow \text{ multiply means and extremes}$$

$$2x = 30$$

Let's try it: Multiply the means and extremes for $2{:}7 = x{:}28$. _____.

 REMEMBER
Always check your answers for accuracy.

means

$$2{:}7 = x{:}28$$

extremes

$$2 \times 28 = 7 \times x$$

9

To determine the value of x, divide both sides of the equation by the number preceding x. Then cancel out like terms. For example:

$$2{:}5 = 6{:}x$$

$$2x = 30 \quad \leftarrow \text{ multiply means and extremes}$$

$$\frac{2x}{2} = \frac{30}{2} \quad \leftarrow \text{ divide by 2}$$

$$\frac{\cancel{2}x}{\cancel{2}} = \frac{\cancel{30}^{15}}{\cancel{2}} \quad \leftarrow \text{ cancel}$$

$$x = 15$$

Practice on this one. Solve for the unknown: $2{:}7 = x{:}28$
$x =$ _____.

$$2{:}7 = x{:}28$$

$$7x = 56$$

$$\frac{7x}{7} = \frac{56}{7}$$

$$\frac{\cancel{7}x}{\cancel{7}} = \frac{\cancel{56}^{8}}{\cancel{7}}$$

$$x = 8$$

———————————————— **10** ————————————————

Always check your answer by substituting it in place of x. The products of the means should equal the products of the extremes. For example:

$$2{:}5 = 6{:}15 \qquad \text{Product of means} = \ \ 30$$
$$\text{Product of extremes} = \ \ 30$$

Now you try one:

$$2{:}7 = 8{:}28 \qquad \text{Product of means} = \text{\_\_\_\_\_}$$
$$\text{Product of extremes} = \text{\_\_\_\_\_}$$

56
56

———————————————— **11** ————————————————

Solve for x in the following proportion: $0.5{:}x = 3{:}6$

$$x = \text{_____}$$

$0.5{:}x = 3{:}6$

$3x = 3$

$\dfrac{3x}{3} = \dfrac{3}{3}$

$x = 1$

 DID YOU NOTICE?

Dividing both sides of the equation by the same number reduces the terms.

———————————————— **12** ————————————————

To prove the answer for the problem, $0.5{:}x = 3{:}6$, substitute _____ for x.

The product of the means = _____.

The product of the extremes = _____.

1

$1 \times 3 = 3$

$0.5 \times 6 = 3$

———————————————— **13** ————————————————

An alternate method used to set up and solve a proportion is to write each ratio as a fraction. Again using the proportion $0.5{:}x = 3{:}6$ as an example, the proportion can be written:

$$\frac{0.5}{x} = \frac{3}{6}$$

To find the product, multiply diagonally. That is, multiply each numerator by the denominator of the fraction across from it. Then solve for the unknown quantity.

$$\frac{0.5}{x} \diagdown \frac{3}{6}$$

$$3x = 3$$

$$\frac{3x}{3} = \frac{3}{3} \quad \longleftarrow \text{ dividing by 3}$$

$$\frac{\cancel{3}x}{\cancel{3}} = \frac{\cancel{3}}{\cancel{3}} \quad \longleftarrow \text{ canceling}$$

$$x = 1$$

Let's try one. Set up the ratios as fractions for the proportion 2:5 = 6:x and solve for x. _____

$$\frac{2}{5} = \frac{6}{x}$$
$$2x = 30$$
$$x = 15$$

The proportion statement expressed as two equal ratios will be used to solve for unknown quantities throughout this book to avoid confusion and errors.

Working with Proportions Containing Fractions

--------------------------------- **14** ---------------------------------

Using ratios and proportions with fractions works equally well. For example:

$$\frac{1}{2} : x = 3:12$$

$$3x = \frac{1}{2} \times \frac{12}{1} \quad \longleftarrow \text{ multiply means and extremes}$$

$$3x = \frac{1}{\cancel{2}} \times \frac{\cancel{12}^{\,6}}{1} \quad \longleftarrow \text{ cancel}$$

$$3x = \frac{6}{1} \quad \longleftarrow \text{ multiply}$$

$$\frac{3x}{3} = \frac{6}{3} \quad \longleftarrow \text{ divide by 3}$$

$$\frac{\cancel{3}x}{\cancel{3}} = \frac{\cancel{6}\,^{2}}{\cancel{3}} \qquad \longleftarrow \text{ cancel}$$

$$x = 2$$

Let's try this problem:

$$3{:}x = \frac{3}{4}{:}2$$

$$x = \underline{\hspace{3cm}}$$

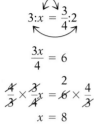

$$3{:}x = \frac{3}{4}{:}2$$

$$\frac{3x}{4} = 6$$

$$\frac{\cancel{4}}{\cancel{3}} \times \frac{\cancel{3}}{\cancel{4}}x = \cancel{6}\,^{2} \times \frac{4}{\cancel{3}}$$

$$x = 8$$

─────────────── **15** ───────────────

Now You Try It

Solve for the unknown quantity in the following proportions.

a. $x{:}\dfrac{1}{2} = 3{:}5 \qquad x = \underline{\hspace{3cm}}$

b. $1{:}\dfrac{1}{5} = 15{:}x \qquad x = \underline{\hspace{3cm}}$

a. $x{:}\dfrac{1}{2} = 3{:}5$

$$5x = \frac{1}{2} \times 3$$

$$5x = 1.5$$

$$\frac{\cancel{5}x}{\cancel{5}} = \frac{\cancel{1.5}\,^{.3}}{\cancel{5}}$$

$$x = 0.3$$

b. $1{:}\dfrac{1}{5} = 15{:}x$

$$x = \frac{1}{\cancel{5}} \times \cancel{15}\,^{3}$$

$$x = 3$$

─────────────── **16** ───────────────

A fraction in a proportion also can be converted to a decimal fraction, before solving for *x*. For example:

$$\frac{3}{5}{:}x = 4{:}7$$

$$0.6{:}x = 4{:}7 \qquad \longleftarrow \text{ change to decimal}$$

$$0.6{:}x = 4{:}7$$

$$4x = 7 \times 0.6 \qquad \longleftarrow \text{ multiply means and extremes}$$

$$4x = 4.2$$

$$\frac{\cancel{A}x}{\cancel{A}} = \frac{\overset{1.05}{\cancel{4.2}}}{\cancel{A}} \quad \longleftarrow \text{cancel}$$

$$x = 1.05$$

DID YOU NOTICE?

Answers should be expressed in whole numbers or decimals. Decimals are more accurate for dosage calculations than fractions.

a. $28:8 = x:0.8$

$8x = 22.4$

$$\frac{\cancel{8}x}{\cancel{8}} = \frac{\overset{2.8}{\cancel{22.4}}}{\cancel{8}}$$

$$x = 2.8$$

17

Now You Try It

Convert the fractions to decimals. Solve for x using the ratio-and-proportion method.

a. $28:8 = x:\dfrac{4}{5}$ $x =$ _____

b. $\dfrac{2}{5}:7 = 3:x$ $x =$ _____

b. $\dfrac{2}{5}:7 = 3:x$

$0.4x = 21$

$$\frac{0.4x}{0.4} = \frac{21}{0.4}$$

$$x = 52.5$$

⭐ What You've Achieved!

★ You can distinguish between the means and the extremes of a proportion.

★ You always remember to place the product containing x on the left side of the equation when solving for an unknown quantity.

★ You can solve for an unknown quantity using the ratio-and-proportion method of calculation.

★ You know how to check your answers for accuracy by substituting the answer for x.

Terrific! The ratio-and-proportion method you've learned to use in this chapter will help you solve all dosage calculation problems. Before moving forward, take the review test to demonstrate your mastery of the subject. If you get more than three wrong, consider studying the chapter again.

Solve for x using the ratio-and-proportion method. Round to the nearest hundredth.

1. $x:3 = 12:9 \quad x =$ _____

2. $7:x = 2:6 \quad x =$ _____

3. $x:3.5 = 24:6 \quad x =$ _____

4. $x:1000 = 7:500 \quad x =$ _____

5. $27:24 = 3:x \quad x =$ _____

6. $7:32 = x:12 \quad x =$ _____

7. $8:x = \frac{2}{5}:7 \quad x =$ _____

8. $x:5 = 0.5:0.25 \quad x =$ _____

9. $\frac{4}{5}:44 = x:11 \quad x =$ _____

10. $0.75:x = 4:80 \quad x =$ _____

11. $4:x = 10:25 \quad x =$ _____

12. $2:7 = 6:x \quad x =$ _____

Answers for Review Test

1. $x:3 = 12:9$
$9x = 36$
$\dfrac{\cancel{9}x}{\cancel{9}} = \dfrac{\cancel{36}^{4}}{\cancel{9}}$
$x = 4$

2. $7:x = 2:6$
$2x = 42$
$\dfrac{\cancel{2}x}{\cancel{2}} = \dfrac{\cancel{42}^{21}}{\cancel{2}}$
$x = 21$

3. $x:3.5 = 24:6$
$6x = 84$
$\dfrac{\cancel{6}x}{\cancel{6}} = \dfrac{\cancel{84}^{14}}{\cancel{6}}$
$x = 14$

4. $x:1000 = 7:500$
$500x = 7000$
$\dfrac{\cancel{500}x}{\cancel{500}} = \dfrac{\cancel{7000}^{14}}{\cancel{500}}$
$x = 14$

---

5. $27:24 = 3:x$
$27x = 72$
$\dfrac{\cancel{27}x}{\cancel{27}} = \dfrac{72}{27}$
$x = 2.67$

6. $7:32 = x:12$
$32x = 84$
$\dfrac{\cancel{32}x}{\cancel{32}} = \dfrac{\cancel{84}^{21}}{\cancel{32}}$
$x = 2.63$

7. $8:x = \dfrac{2}{5}:7$
$\dfrac{2x}{5} = 56$
$\dfrac{\cancel{5}}{\cancel{2}} \times \dfrac{\cancel{2}}{\cancel{5}}x = \cancel{56}^{28} \times \dfrac{5}{\cancel{2}}$
$x = 28 \times 5$
$x = 140$

$8:x = \dfrac{2}{5}:7$

$8:x = 0.4:7$
$0.4x = 56$
$\dfrac{\cancel{0.4}x}{\cancel{0.4}} = \dfrac{56}{0.4}$
$x = 140$

8. $x{:}5 = .5{:}.25$

$0.25x = 2.5$

$$\frac{0.25x}{0.25} = \frac{2.5}{0.25}^{\,10}$$

$x = 10$

9. $\dfrac{4}{5}{:}44 = x{:}11$

$44x = \dfrac{4}{5} \times 11$

$44x = \dfrac{44}{5}$

$$\frac{44x}{44} = \frac{8.8}{44}^{\,0.2}$$

$x = 0.2$

$\dfrac{4}{5}{:}44 = x{:}11$

$0.8{:}44 = x{:}11$

$44x = 8.8$

$$\frac{44x}{44} = \frac{8.8}{44}^{\,0.2}$$

$x = 0.2$

10. $0.75{:}x = 4{:}80$

$4x = 60$

$$\frac{4x}{4} = \frac{60}{4}^{\,15}$$

$x = 15$

11. $4{:}x = 10{:}25$

$10x = 100$

$$\frac{10x}{10} = \frac{100}{10}^{\,10}$$

$x = 10$

12. $2{:}7 = 6{:}x$

$2x = 42$

$$\frac{2x}{2} = \frac{42}{2}^{\,21}$$

$x = 21$

II

SYSTEMS OF MEASUREMENT FOR DOSAGE CALCULATIONS

 HEALTH CARE PROFESSIONALS IN THE United States use three systems of weighing and measuring drugs. They are the metric system, the apothecary system, and the household system.

Most European countries and Canada require the use of the metric system for prescribing dosages. In the United States, however, the apothecary system is still used to dispense some medication preparations. Moreover, the household system of measurement is actually gaining in importance as the delivery of health care shifts to the home, where patients and nurses depend on teaspoons and other common household containers to measure drugs.

Understanding all three systems of measurement and developing the skills necessary to convert from one system to another is essential for accurately calculating drug dosages or for preparing and administering medications. This section will introduce you to these three systems of measurement. You will also use the ratio-and-proportion method to convert measurements between the three systems.

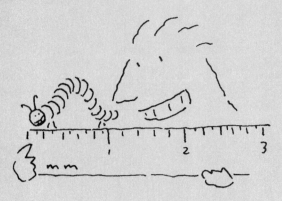

The Metric System

5

Objectives

When you finish this chapter, you will be able to:

★ Name the basic units of measurement in the metric system.

★ Identify abbreviations commonly used in the metric system.

★ Use the correct notation rules to express metric weights and volumes.

★ Convert metric weights from one unit of measurement to another.

★ Convert metric volumes between liters and milliliters.

Chapter Outline

★ Basic Metric Units of Measurement

★ Multiples and Subdivisions of Metric Units

★ Numeric Values of Metric Multiples and Subdivisions

★ Expressing Metric Quantities

★ Converting Between Metric Units of Measurement

★ Shortcut for Converting Between Equivalent Metric Units

Introduction

The **metric system** of weights and measures is the system of choice when calculating drug dosages. Based on the decimal system, the metric system arranges units of weights and measures according to multiples and divisions of ten. The basic metric units of measurement are the **gram** (weight or mass), the **liter** (volume or liquid quantity), and the **meter** (length or linear measurement). Table 5.1 shows the basic metric units. Metric prefixes indicate multiples or subdivisions of these basic units. You will use weight and volume measurements frequently when calculating drug dosages.

TABLE 5.1 **Basic Metric Units of Measurement**

Measurement	Unit	Abbreviation
weight (mass)	gram	g
volume (liquid quantity)	liter	L
length (linear measurement)	meter	m

Basic Metric Units of Measurement

1

The system of measurement that is most often used when calculating drug dosages is the _____ _____.

metric system

2

The metric system is based on the decimal system and uses units of measurement that are multiples or divisions of _____.

10

3

The gram is the basic unit of _____ in the metric system.

weight (mass)

4

The liter is the basic unit of liquid _____ in the metric system.

volume

5

Metric units of measurement are commonly written in abbreviated form. Official abbreviations are derived from the first letter of each unit's name and are written in lowercase letters. An exception is the use of a capital "L" to designate liters. You might encounter some older unofficial abbreviations for the gram (Gm and gm) and liter (l). These are still used on some drug labels.

Remember, the preferred abbreviation for the gram is _____.

g

---------------------------- **6** ----------------------------

The preferred abbreviation for liter is _____.

L

Multiples and Subdivisions of Metric Units

---------------------------- **7** ----------------------------

Prefixes, when combined with the basic unit names, indicate the
_____ or _____ of the basic units. Table 5.2
illustrates the prefixes and their numerical value for the subdivisions and multiples of any basic metric unit. You will use only the
prefixes **kilo-**, **milli-**, and **micro-** when calculating drug dosages.

subdivisions
multiples

TABLE 5.2 **Metric Prefixes and Numerical Values**

	Prefix	Abbreviation	Numerical Value	
multiples	*kilo	k	1000	(one thousand)
	hecto	h	100	(one hundred)
	deka	dk	10	(ten)
	Basic Metric Units			
	deci	d	0.1	(one-tenth)
	centi	c	0.01	(one-hundredth)
	*milli	m	0.001	(one-thousandth)
subdivisions	*micro	mc	0.000001	(one-millionth)

---------------------------- **8** ----------------------------

In the metric system, the prefix indicates the multiple or subdivi-
sion of _____.

the basic unit

---------------------------- **9** ----------------------------

You indicate multiples and subdivisions of the basic units of
weight (_____) and volume (_____) by writing
a prefix before the name of the basic unit.

gram
liter

---------------------------- **10** ----------------------------

The **kilogram** is the only multiple of the gram used to calculate
drug dosages and represents a _____ that is larger than
the gram.

weight

---- **11** ----

The two most common subdivisions of the gram used to calculate drug dosages are the **milligram** and **microgram**. Micrograms and milligrams represent weights that are ＿＿＿＿＿＿＿ than the gram.

less

---- **12** ----

Milli- is the only prefix you will use with the liter. Milli- indicates a volume that is less than the liter and is written as ＿＿＿＿＿.

milliliter

---- **13** ----

The abbreviations for multiples and subdivisions of metric units are derived from the prefix and the unit names. (See Table 5.2.) For example, the abbreviation for kilogram is kg.

Now you write the abbreviation for milligram, ＿＿＿＿＿＿.

mg

---- **14** ----

One variation you might notice on occasion is the abbreviation for microgram. You may see the symbol μ on some medication labels to indicate the prefix micro-. However, use mc to represent micro- to assure accurate interpretation of drug amounts. Remember, the preferred abbreviation for microgram is ＿＿＿＿.

mcg

---- **15** ----

Another exception you may encounter is the abbreviation for milliliter. An unofficial abbreviation for milliliter is written entirely in lowercase letters as ml. Remember, the official base unit abbreviation is a capital letter. You should write milliliter as ＿＿＿＿＿.

mL

---- **16** ----

A **cubic centimeter** is the amount of space one milliliter of liquid occupies. One cubic centimeter is equivalent to one milliliter. The practice of substituting mL for ＿＿＿ is a common occurrence.

cc

Now You Try It

Write the correct abbreviations for the following metric units of measures.

a. microgram   = _____   a. mcg

b. milligram   = _____   b. mg

c. gram   = _____   c. g

d. kilogram   = _____   d. kg

e. milliliter   = _____   e. mL

f. cubic centimeter = _____ f. cc

g. liter   = _____   g. L

Numeric Values of Metric Multiples and Subdivisions

18

Prefixes indicate a change in the numeric value of the basic unit. Kilo- indicates a numeric value 1000 times **greater** than the basic unit, while milli- indicates a numerical value 1000 times **smaller** than the basic unit. Micro- indicates a numerical value 1,000,000 times **smaller** than the basic unit and 1000 times **smaller** than the milli- unit. Using this principle, 1 kilogram is equal to _____ grams.   1000

REMEMBER

You will not calculate drug dosages using decimals smaller than 0.001.

19

One milligram is equal to one-thousandth (0.001) of a gram, while one gram is equal to _____ milligrams.   1000

20

1,000,000

One microgram is equal to one-millionth (0.000001) of a gram, while _____ micrograms are equal to one gram.

21

1000

One microgram is equal to one-thousandth (0.001) of a milligram, while one milligram is equal to _____ micrograms.

REMEMBER

Metric prefixes indicate multiples or subdivisions of basic metric units. This figure illustrates the relationship of all prefixes to the basic unit.

Metric Prefixes

kilo-	hecto-	deka-	basic metric unit	deci-	centi-	milli-	micro-
1000	100	10	0	0.1	0.01	0.001	0.000001

22

Try this example:

0.001
1000

One milliliter is equal to _____ liter, while one liter is equal to _____ milliliters.

23

Now You Try It

Determine the numeric value of the following metric measurements.

a. 1000   **a.** 1 g   = _____ mg

b. 1   **b.** 1000 mg = _____ g

c. 1000   **c.** 1 kg   = _____ g

d. 1   **d.** 1000 g = _____ kg

e. 1000   **e.** 1 L   = _____ cc

f. 1 cc $\quad$ = _____ mL

g. 1000 mL = _____ L

h. 1000 mcg = _____ mg

i. 1 mg $\quad$ = _____ mcg

f. 1

g. 1

h. 1

i. 1000

REMEMBER

One milliliter (mL) is equivalent to one cubic centimeter (cc). The practice of substituting the abbreviation mL for cc is a common occurrence.

Expressing Metric Quantities

24

Follow three rules of notation when expressing quantities in the metric system.

Rule 1 Express numbers in the Arabic numbering system (such as 1, 2, and 3) and write the numbers before the abbreviation of metric units. For example:

$$5 \text{ g}$$

Rule 2 Use decimals to represent fractional amounts of a number. For example, one and one-half grams is written as:

$$1.5 \text{ g}$$

Rule 3 Write a zero as a placeholder in front of a decimal point when it is not preceded by a whole number. For example:

$$0.5 \text{ g}$$

Applying these rules, you would write one-third of a gram (rounded to the nearest tenth) as _____.

0.3 g

REMEMBER

If necessary, refresh your understanding of decimals by rereading Chapter 3, frames 1 through 12.

---- **25** ----

Now You Try It

Write the following metric weights and volumes using the correct notation rules and abbreviations. Round decimal numbers to the nearest hundredth.

a. 4 kg

b. 50 mL

c. 0.67 mcg

d. 1.25 L

e. 300 cc

f. 5.7 g

g. 800 mg

a. four kilograms _____

b. fifty milliliters _____

c. two-thirds microgram _____

d. one and one-fourth liter _____

e. three hundred cubic centimeters _____

f. five and seven-tenths grams _____

g. eight hundred milligrams _____

Converting Between Metric Units of Measurement

---- **26** ----

When calculating drug dosages prescribed in the metric system, it may be necessary to convert between multiples and subdivisions of a unit of metric measurement. To do this, you need only remember the basic units of measurement, the meaning of the prefixes, and how to use ratios and proportions to solve for an unknown quantity, represented by the letter _____.

x

To use the ratio-and-proportion method to convert between metric equivalents, we begin with a known ratio between two units, such as grams and milligrams or liters and milliliters. To make sure the proportion is set up correctly, follow a three-step process.

---- **27** ----

First, write a proportion showing the "known ratio" on the left and the "want-to-know" ratio, containing the unknown quantity, on the right.

known
want-to-know

"_____" ratio = "_____ ____ _____" ratio

--- **28** ---

Second, rewrite the proportion using the units to be converted. The sequence of units must be the same in both ratios. For example

g:mg = g:mg OR mg:g = mg:g, NOT g:mg = mg:g

Now substitute the numeric values for the units of the known ratio on the left and the want-to-know ratio on the right. Use x for the unknown quantity. For example, suppose you want to convert 425 milligrams into grams. Since 1 gram equals _____ milligrams, the known ratio is 1:1000. For the want-to-know ratio, we already know the quantity in milligrams; x stands for the quantity in grams, which we do not yet know.

1000

1:1000 = x:425

--- **29** ---

Third, multiply the _____ and _____ and solve for x. Remember to label the answer with the correct unit of metric measurement to avoid errors.

means
extremes

Now let's put the three steps together to convert 425 milligrams to grams:

known = want-to-know

g:mg = g:mg ⟵ **proportion in metric units**

1:1000 = x:425 ⟵ **proportion with numeric values**

1:1000 = x:425 ⟵ **multiply means and extremes**

1000x = 425

$\dfrac{1000x}{1000}$ = $\dfrac{425}{1000}$ ⟵ **cancel**

x = 0.425

Therefore, 425 mg = 0.425 g.

known = want-to-know
g:mg = g:mg
1:1000 = 2.3:x

1:1000 = 2.3:x

x = 2300
2.3 g = 2300 mg

--- **30** ---

Now practice with this one. Convert 2.3 g to an equivalent number of milligrams: 2.3 g = _____ mg

REMEMBER

You may want to review Chapter 4, frames 8 through 12, to refresh your understanding of ratios and proportions.

————————————————— **31** —————————————————

Let's try an example:

Your patient is to receive 1500 milliliters of water. How many liters is this? _____

$$L{:}mL = L{:}mL \quad \longleftarrow \text{ proportion in metric units}$$

$$1{:}1000 = x{:}1500 \quad \longleftarrow \text{ numeric values}$$

$$1{:}1000 = x{:}1500 \quad \longleftarrow \text{ multiply means and extremes}$$

$$1000x = 1500$$

$$\frac{1000x}{1000} = \frac{1500}{1000} \quad \longleftarrow \text{ cancel}$$

$$x = 1.5$$

Therefore, 1500 mL = 1.5 L.

————————————————— **32** —————————————————

Try this problem: A premature infant weighs 880 grams. Figure the weight in kilograms.

$$880 \text{ g} = \underline{\hspace{2cm}} \text{ kg}$$

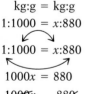

kg:g = kg:g
1:1000 = x:880

1:1000 = x:880

1000x = 880

$\frac{1000x}{1000} = \frac{880}{1000}$

x = 0.88
880 g = 0.88 kg

REMEMBER

Use metric equivalents to create the "known" ratio when converting from one metric unit to another metric unit.

Equivalent Metric Measurements

Metric Weights

1 kg	=	1000 g
1 g	=	1000 mg
1 mg	=	1000 mcg

Metric Volumes

$$1 \text{ L} = 1000 \text{ mL (cc)}$$
$$1 \text{ mL} = 1 \text{ cc}$$

— 33 —

Now You Try It

Convert the following metric equivalents using the ratio and proportion method.

a. 4.2 kg = _____ g

b. 0.5 L = _____ cc

c. 3.25 mg = _____ mcg

d. 75 mg = _____ g

e. Your patient drinks 750 mL of water over 8 hours. How many liters is this? _____

f. Your patient receives 180 mcg of a drug. Convert this to milligrams. _____

 DID YOU NOTICE?

Most calculations of metric equivalents are derived by simply multiplying or dividing by 1000.

Shortcut for Converting Between Equivalent Metric Units

— 34 —

The numeric values for kilogram, gram, milligram, and microgram, and for liter and milliliter differ by 1000 between each increment. You will only calculate drug dosages by one increment. Knowing this fact, you can use a shortcut to convert between the metric units of measurement. To use the shortcut, simply move the decimal point three places to the **right** when converting a **larger** unit of measurement to the next equivalent

a.   kg:g = kg:g

1:1000 = 4.2:*x*

x = 4,200 g

b.   L:cc = L:cc

1:1000 = 0.5:*x*

x = 500 cc

c. mg:mcg = mg:mcg

1:1000 = 3.25:*x*

x = 3,250 mcg

d.   mg:g = mg:g

1000:1 = 75:*x*

1000*x* = 75

$$\frac{1000x}{1000} = \frac{75}{1000}$$

x = 0.075 g

e.   mL:L = mL:L

1000:1 = 750:*x*

1000*x* = 750

$$\frac{1000x}{1000} = \frac{750}{1000}$$

x = 0.75 L

f. mcg:mg = mcg:mg

1000:1 = 180:*x*

1000*x* = 180

$$\frac{1000x}{1000} = \frac{180}{1000}$$

x = 0.18 mg

smaller unit of measurement. For example, let's convert 8 kilograms to an equivalent measurement in grams:

$$8 \text{ kg} = \underline{\quad ? \quad} \text{ g}$$

$$8.\underset{1\ 2\ 3}{0\,0\,0}. = 8000$$

$$8 \text{ kg} = 8000 \text{ g}$$

8 kilograms is equivalent to 8000 grams.

Try converting 0.25 grams to an equivalent measurement in milligrams:

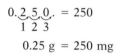

$$0.\underset{1\ 2\ 3}{2\,5\,0}. = 250$$

$$0.25 \text{ g} = 250 \text{ mg}$$

$$0.25 \text{ g} = \underline{\hspace{2cm}} \text{ mg}$$

DID YOU NOTICE?

Moving the decimal point three places to the right produces the same answer as multiplying by 1000.

── **35** ──

Conversely, to convert a **smaller** unit of metric measurement to the next equivalent **larger** unit of metric measurement, move the decimal point three places to the **left**. For example, let's convert 600 milligrams to an equivalent measurement in grams:

$$600 \text{ mg} = \underline{\quad ? \quad} \text{ g}$$

$$600. \underset{3\ 2\ 1}{} = 0.6$$

$$600 \text{ mg} = 0.6 \text{ g}$$

600 milligrams is equivalent to 0.6 grams.

Now, you convert 5500 micrograms to an equivalent measurement of milligrams:

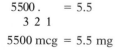

$$5500. \underset{3\ 2\ 1}{} = 5.5$$

$$5500 \text{ mcg} = 5.5 \text{ mg}$$

$$5500 \text{ mcg} = \underline{\hspace{1.5cm}} \text{ mg}$$

DID YOU NOTICE?

Moving the decimal point three places to the left produces the same answer as dividing by 1000.

Now You Try It

Convert the following metric measurements using the shortcut.

a. 5 g   = _____ mg

b. 1.39 L   = _____ mL

c. 0.065 mg = _____ mcg

d. 600 mcg = _____ mg

e. 125 cc   = _____ L

f. 40 g   = _____ kg

a. 5.0 0 0. = 5000
    1 2 3

     5 g = 5000 mg

b. 1.3 9 0. = 1390
    1 2 3

    1.39 L = 1390 mL

c. 0.0 6 5. = 65
    1 2 3

   0.065 mg = 65 mcg

d. 600 . = 0.6
    3 2 1

   600 mcg = 0.6 mg

e. 125 . = 0.125
    3 2 1

   125 cc = 0.125 L

f. . 40 . = 0.04
   3 2 1

    40 g = 0.04 kg

☆ **What You've Achieved!**

★ You've learned the basic units of measurement in the metric system.

★ You know how to express metric weights and volumes using correct notation rules and abbreviations.

★ You can convert metric equivalents using the ratio-and-proportion method.

Great work! What you've learned in this chapter will help you in calculating drug dosages prescribed in the metric system. Before moving forward, take the review test to demonstrate your mastery of the metric system. If you get more than one wrong in any section, consider rereading that portion of the chapter.

Review Test

A

Indicate whether the statements are true or false. If false, correct the statement.

1. _____ The gram is the basic unit of weight in the metric system.

2. _____ The milliliter is the basic unit of volume in the metric system.

3. _____ A milligram is a unit of weight.

4. _____ A cubic centimeter is a unit of weight.

5. _____ In the metric system, fractional drug dosages will be expressed as common fractions.

B

Express the following metric weights and volumes using correct notation rules and abbreviations.

6. Two grams _____

7. Five hundred cubic centimeters _____

8. One-half liter _____

9. Two-tenths milligram _____

10. Five-hundredths gram _____

11. Two and one-half kilograms _____

12. One hundred micrograms _____

13. Two and three-tenths milliliter _____

C

Convert the following metric equivalents using the ratio-and-proportion method.

14. 900 mcg = _____ mg

15. 500 g = _____ kg

16. 3750 mL = _____ L

D

Solve the following word problems.

17. The medication order reads Keflex, 250 milligrams. How many grams is this? _____

18. The doctor orders Digoxin, 0.125 milligrams. Convert the value to micrograms. _____

19. Your patient is to receive Lopid, 0.3 grams. Calculate the quantity in milligrams. _____

20. You are to administer Maalox, 15 milliliters. How many cubic centimeters is this? _____

21. The patient's intake is 2.1 liters of fluid. How many cubic centimeters is this? _____

22. A newborn weighs 2.5 kilograms. Figure the weight in grams. _____

Answers for Review Test

1. T	**2.** F, liter	**3.** T	**4.** F, volume	**5.** F, decimals

6. 2 g	**7.** 500 cc	**8.** 0.5 L	**9.** 0.2 mg	**10.** 0.05 g

11. 2.5 kg	**12.** 100 mcg	**13.** 2.3 mL

14. mcg:mg = mcg:mg

$$1000:1 = 900:x$$

$$1000x = 900$$

$$\frac{1000x}{1000} = \frac{900}{1000}$$

$$x = 0.9 \text{ mg}$$

15. g:kg = g:kg

$$1000:1 = 500:x$$

$$1000x = 500$$

$$\frac{1000x}{1000} = \frac{500}{1000}$$

$$x = 0.5 \text{ kg}$$

16. mL:L = mL:L

$$1000:1 = 3750:x$$

$$1000x = 3750$$

$$\frac{1000x}{1000} = \frac{3750}{1000}$$

$$x = 3.75 \text{ L}$$

17. g:mg = g:mg

$$1:1000 = x:250$$

$$1000x = 250$$

$$\frac{1000x}{1000} = \frac{250}{1000}$$

$$x = .25 \text{ g}$$

18. mg:mcg = mg:mcg

$$1:1000 = 0.125:x$$

$$x = 125 \text{ mcg}$$

19. g:mg = g:mg

$$1:1000 = 0.3:x$$

$$x = 300 \text{ mg}$$

20. 15 mL = 15 cc

21. L:cc = L:cc

$$1:1000 = 2.1:x$$

$$x = 2100 \text{ cc}$$

22. kg:g = kg:g

$$1:1000 = 2.5:x$$

$$x = 2500 \text{ g}$$

6

The Apothecary System

Objectives

When you finish this chapter, you will be able to:

★ Name the basic units of the apothecary system.

★ Write the abbreviations commonly used in the apothecary system.

★ Use correct notation rules to express apothecary weights and volumes.

★ Convert apothecary volumes from one unit of measure to another.

Chapter Outline

★ Basic Apothecary Units of Measurement

★ Expressing Apothecary Quantities

★ Numeric Value of Apothecary Units

★ Converting Between Apothecary Units of Measurement

Introduction

The **apothecary system** of measurement, adopted by the American colonists, is slowly being replaced by the metric system. It is used in a limited manner by physicians to prescribe medications that have been in use for a long period of time, such as aspirin. The apothecary system uses Roman numerals for small quantities of the unit, and fractions for parts of a whole unit. The basic unit of weight is the **grain** (gr), while the **minim** (♏) is the basic unit of volume. Table 6.1 shows the apothecary units of measure and abbreviations. You will use minims, fluidrams, fluidounces, and grains when calculating drug dosages in the apothecary system.

TABLE 6.1 Basic Units of Measurement

Measurement	Unit	Abbreviations
weight	grain	gr
	pound	lb
volume	minim	ℳ
	fluidram	f℥
	fluidounce	f℥
	pint	pt

Basic Apothecary Units of Measurement

1

The _____ _____ is the system of measurement that is slowly being phased out by the metric system.

apothecary system

2

The grain is the basic unit of _____ and is defined as the weight of an average sized grain of wheat.

weight

3

The _____ is the basic unit of volume in the apothecary system. It is equivalent to the quantity of water that weighs a grain and is approximately the size of a drop of water.

minim

4

Apothecary units of measurement are commonly written in abbreviated form. The grain is the only unit of weight used. You will use the grain when calculating dosage conversions between the metric and apothecary systems. You write the abbreviation for grain as _____.

gr

DID YOU NOTICE?

The grain is abbreviated gr to avoid confusion with the abbreviation for gram, g.

5

The official abbreviation for the **dram** is ℨ and the **ounce** is ℥. Place an "f" in front of the abbreviations for dram and ounce to correctly express fluidram and fluidounce. Physicans sometimes drop the "f" however, and write orders for **fluidram** as ℨ and **fluidounce** as ℥. You will use the symbols fℨ and f℥ throughout this book. Remember, the preferred abbreviation for fluidounce is _____.

f℥

> DID YOU NOTICE?
> The smaller unit, fluidram, contains one loop in its abbreviation, ℨ, while the larger unit, fluidounce, contains two loops in its abbreviation ℥.

6
---

f℥

Now, write the abbreviation for fluidram, _____.

7

℔

The minim, which is the basic liquid quantity, is abbreviated by ℔. You may see an alternate abbreviation written as m. You will write the preferred abbreviation for minim as _____.

8

Now You Try It

Write the correct abbreviation for the following apothecary units of measure.

a. lb

b. fℨ

c. f℥

d. ℔

e. gr

a. pound   = _____

b. fluidram   = _____

c. fluidounce = _____

d. minim   = _____

e. grain   = _____

Expressing Apothecary Quantities

9

The abbreviation precedes the amount when expressing apothecary quantities. Smaller quantities (less than 30) are expressed as Roman numerals. The abbreviation for 15 minims is _____.

℩ XV

 REMEMBER

Write numerical values of 30 or less in the apothecary system as Roman numerals. Use Arabic numbers to calculate all apothecary drug dosages. Review Chapter 1 to refresh your understanding of number systems.

10

One variation you might notice is the abbreviation ss, used to represent the number one-half. It is written after the quantity. For instance, eight and one-half fluidrams is written as f℥ VIIIss.

You write nine and one-half fluidounces as _____.

f℥ IXss

11

Except where the fraction is $\frac{1}{2}$, dosage quantities of other than whole numbers are written entirely in Arabic using fractions. For example, two-thirds of a minim is written as ℩ $\frac{2}{3}$.

Now try this. Write the abbreviation for three quarters of a grain. _____

gr $\frac{3}{4}$

12

Now You Try It

Write the following apothecary weights and volumes using the correct notation rules and abbreviations.

a. four fluidounces _____

a. f℥ IV

b. one-half minim _____

b. ℩ ss

c. gr XXX

d. f℥ IX

e. fℨ VIII

f. lb X

g. pts XVII

h. fℨ $3\frac{1}{3}$

c. thirty grains _____

d. nine fluidounces _____

e. eight fluidrams _____

f. ten pounds _____

g. seventeen pints _____

h. three and one-third fluidram _____

Numeric Value of Apothecary Units

— **13** —

You need to know the numeric value of the apothecary units to convert between units of measurement in the apothecary system. You need only learn two equivalents for apothecary volumes:

1. 60 minims are equal to one fluidram;

2. 8 fluidrams are equal to one fluidounce.

grain

Remember, no conversion between apothecary weights is necessary because the _____ is the only unit of weight used.

— **14** —

60

Let's review. One fluidram is equal to _____ minims.

— **15** —

8

Now try this equivalent. One fluidounce is equal to _____ fluidrams.

Converting Between Apothecary Units of Measurement

— **16** —

Use the ratio-and-proportion method for converting between units of measurement in the apothecary system. Remember, the basic method involves three steps. First, select two equal ratios and write them as a proportion. The ratio on the left side of the proportion represents the "_____" ratio of apothecary equivalents. The ratio on the right side of the proportion represents the "_____ _____ _____" ratio.

known

want-to-know

―――――――――――― **17** ――――――――――――

Second, write down the units in proportional form and then the quantities in proportional form. Third, multiply the means and extremes and solve for the unknown quantity. For example, let's convert 15 minims to fluidrams:

known = want-to-know

$\text{m}:\text{f}\mathfrak{z} = \text{m}:\text{f}\mathfrak{z}$ ⟵ **proportion in apothecary units**

$60:1 = 15:x$ ⟵ **proportion with numeric values**

$60:1 = 15:x$ ⟵ **multiply means and extremes**

$60x = 15$

$$\frac{\cancel{60}x}{\cancel{60}} = \frac{\overset{1}{\cancel{15}}}{\underset{4}{\cancel{60}}}$$ ⟵ **cancel**

$$x = \frac{1}{4}$$

Therefore, 15 minims are equivalent to one-quarter fluidram or $\text{m} \, XV = \text{f}\mathfrak{z} \, \frac{1}{4}$.

 REMEMBER

Reread Chapter 4 if you need to review your understanding of the ratio-and-proportion method.

$\text{f}\mathfrak{z}:\text{f}\mathfrak{z} = \text{f}\mathfrak{z}:\text{f}\mathfrak{z}$

$1:8 = \frac{3}{4}:x$

$1:8 = \frac{3}{4}:x$

$$x = \frac{\overset{6}{\cancel{24}}}{\cancel{4}}$$

$x = \text{f}\mathfrak{z} \, VI$

$\text{f}\mathfrak{z} \, \frac{3}{4} = \text{f}\mathfrak{z} \, VI$

―――――――――――― **18** ――――――――――――

Now you try this one. Convert $\text{f}\mathfrak{z} \, \frac{3}{4}$ to $\text{f}\mathfrak{z}$. _____

 REMEMBER

Use Apothecary equivalents when converting from one apothecary volume to another.

Equivalents for Apothecary Units of Volume

60 minims (♏) = 1 fluidram (f℥)
480 minims (♏) = 8 fluidrams (℥) = 1 fluidounce (℥)
16 fluidounces (f℥) = 1 pint (pt)
---

a. ♏:f℥ = ♏:f℥

480:1 = 240:x

480x = 240

$x = f℥ \frac{1}{2}$ (ss)

b. f℥:f℥ = f℥:f℥

1:8 = 2.5:x

x = 20

x = f℥ XX

c. f℥:♏ = f℥:♏

1:480 = 1.5:x

x = ♏ 720

d. f℥:f℥ = f℥:f℥

8:1 = 16:x

8x = 16

$\frac{8x}{8} = \frac{\overset{2}{\cancel{16}}}{\cancel{8}}$

x = f℥ II

19

Now You Try It

Convert the following apothecary equivalents using the ratio and proportion method.

a. 240 minims = f℥ _____

b. f℥ IIss = f℥ _____

c. f℥ Iss = ♏ _____

d. f℥ XVI = f℥ _____

☆ **What You've Achieved!**

★ You know the basic units of the apothecary system.

★ You always remember to express apothecary weights and volumes using correct notation rules and abbreviations.

★ You know how to convert apothecary volumes from one unit of measure to another.

Terrific! What you've achieved in this unit will help you convert between apothecary units. Before moving on to the next chapter, take the review test to demonstrate your mastery of the apothecary system. If you get more than one question wrong in any section, consider studying that portion of the chapter again.

―――――――――――――――――――――――― **A** ――――――――――――――――――――――――

Indicate whether the statement is true or false. If it is false, correct the underlined term of the statements.

1. _____ The <u>minim</u> designates a liquid quantity.

2. _____ The <u>dram</u> is the basic unit of weight in the apothecary system.

3. _____ Fractional drug dosages are expressed as <u>decimals</u> in the apothecary system.

4. _____ Roman numerals are used to express <u>large</u> quantities in the apothecary system.

5. _____ <u>Arabic</u> numbers are used when solving dosage problems in the apothecary system.

―――――――――――――――――――――――― **B** ――――――――――――――――――――――――

Express the following apothecary weights and volumes using correct notation rules and abbreviations.

6. twenty and one-half grains _____

7. eight pounds _____

8. nineteen pints _____

9. two and one-half fluidrams _____

10. six and five-eighths fluidounces _____

11. fourteen minims _____

12. twenty-four fluidounces _____

―――――――――――――――――――――――― **C** ――――――――――――――――――――――――

Convert the following apothecary equivalents using the ratio and proporation method.

13. ℥ 90 = f℥ _____

14. f℥ ss = ℥ _____

15. f℥ VIIss = ℥ _____

16. f℥ $1\frac{1}{4}$ = f℥ _____

17. ℥ 180 = f℥ _____

18. f℥ IV = f℥ _____

19. The physician orders Ensure, f℥ 4. How many fʒ is this? _____

20. The patient is to receive M.O.M. fʒ 16. Convert this to f℥. _____

Answers for Review Test

1. T	**2.** F, grain	**3.** F, fractions	**4.** F, small	**5.** T

6. gr XXss	**7.** lb VIII	**8.** pt XIX	**9.** fʒ IIss	**10.** f℥ $6\frac{5}{8}$

11. ♏ XIV   **12.** f℥ XXIV

13. f℥:♏ = f℥:♏

$$1:480 = x:90$$

$$\frac{480x}{480} = \frac{90}{480}$$

$$x = \text{f℥}\ \frac{3}{16}$$

14. ♏:f℥ = ♏:f℥

$$60:1 = x:0.5$$

$$x = \text{♏}\ 30\ (\text{♏ XXX})$$

15. f℥:♏ = f℥:♏

$$1:480 = 7.5:x$$

$$x = \text{♏}\ 3600$$

16. f℥:fʒ = f℥:fʒ

$$1:8 = 1.25:x$$

$$x = \text{fʒ}\ 10\ (\text{fʒ X})$$

17. f℥:♏ = f℥:♏

$$1:60 = x:180$$

$$\frac{60x}{60} = \frac{180}{60}$$

$$x = \text{f℥ III}$$

18. f℥:fʒ = f℥:fʒ

$$1:8 = x:4$$

$$\frac{8x}{8} = \frac{4}{8}$$

$$x = \text{f℥ ss}$$

19. f℥:fʒ = f℥:fʒ

$$1:8 = 4:x$$

$$x = \text{fʒ}\ 32$$

20. f℥:fʒ = f℥:fʒ

$$8:1 = 16:x$$

$$\frac{8x}{8} = \frac{\overset{2}{16}}{8}$$

$$x = \text{f℥}\ 2\ (\text{f℥ II})$$

The Household System and Dosages Measured in Units and Milliequivalents

7

Objectives

When you finish this chapter, you will be able to:

★ Name the basic liquid units of the household system.

★ Define unit and milliequivalent.

★ Write the abbreviations commonly used in the household system.

★ Write the abbreviations used for units and milliequivalents.

★ Convert household volumes from one unit of measure to another unit of measure.

Chapter Outline

★ Household Units of Measurement

★ Numeric Values for Household Measurements

★ Converting Between Household Units of Measurement

★ Units and Milliequivalents

Introduction

Household System

The **household system** of measurement is used at home by patients when self-administering liquid medications. The household system is less accurate than the metric or apothecary systems of measurement because the containers used may vary in size from household to household. Health care settings only use these units of measurement when a standard calibrated medication receptacle (a plastic medicine cup) is available to provide a more accurate dosage. The common household measures for volume include **drops** (gtt), **teaspoons** (t or tsp), and **tablespoons** (T or tbs).

Units and Milliequivalents

Two other notations, **units** (U) and **milliequivalents** (mEq), may be used when prescribing dosages of certain drugs. Both measures indicate the potency or strength that causes specific therapeutic effect from the prescribed medication. You will not perform conversion problems for units or milliequivalents.

Household Units of Measurement

1

The household system is the least accurate system of measurement because the measuring container sizes vary from household to household. You will use a _____ _____ _____ in health care settings to provide a more accurate measurement of medication.

calibrated medication receptacle

2

The most common units of household liquid measures are the _____ and _____.

teaspoon
tablespoon

3

No standard notation rules exist for the household system. Therefore the abbreviation may precede or follow the dosage amount. For example:

5 tsp *or* tsp 5

For ease of reading, write the numeric value in Arabic numbers followed by the abbreviation. You will express three tablespoons as _____ or _____.

3 T
3 tbs

4

Now You Try It

Write the following household units using correct abbreviations.

a. eight tablespoons _____ or _____

b. twenty-four drops _____

c. eleven teaspoons _____ or _____

a. 8 T or 8 tbs

b. 24 gtts

c. 11 t or 11 tsp

REMEMBER

Use a lowercase t for the smaller quantity, teaspoon, and a capital T for the larger quantity, tablespoon.

Numeric Values for Household Measurements

5

You need to know the numeric value of the units in the household system in order to convert between units. Table 7.1 provides a summary of household measurements.

TABLE 7.1 **Household Units of Measurement**

Measure	Abbreviation	Equivalents
1 drop	gtt	1 minim
1 teaspoon	t or tsp	60 drops
1 tablespoon	T or tbs	3 teaspoons
1 ounce	f℥	2 tablespoons

You should consider the equivalents as only approximate estimates. For instance, one drop is approximately equal to one _____.

minim

DID YOU NOTICE?

The household measure for ounce is the same as that of the apothecary fluidounce.

6

60

Now let's review. One teaspoon is equal to _____ drops.

7

2

One ounce equals _____ tablespoons.

8

3

One tablespoon is equal to _____ teaspoons.

Converting Between Household Units of Measurement

9
---

unknown

Use the ratio-and-proportion method to convert between household units of measure. To review, first select two equal ratios and write them as a proportion, labeled "known" ratio and "want-to-know" ratio. Next, write the units in proportional form and then write the quantities in proportional form. Finally, multiply the means and the extremes and solve for the _____ quantity. For example, let's convert 7 teaspoons to tablespoons:

known ratio = want-to-know ratio

tbs:tsp = tbs:tsp ⟵ proportion in units

$1:3 = x:7$ ⟵ proportion with numeric values

$1:3 = x:7$ ⟵ multiply means and extremes

$3x = 7$

$\dfrac{\cancel{3}x}{\cancel{3}} = \dfrac{7}{3}$ ⟵ cancel

$x = 2\dfrac{1}{3} \text{ tbs}$

Therefore, 7 teaspoons is equivalent to $2\frac{1}{3}$ tablespoons (7 tsp = $2\frac{1}{3}$ tbs).

Practice on this one. Convert $\frac{2}{3}$ teaspoon to drops.

_____

REMEMBER

Use household equivalents when converting between units of volume measures.

Household Equivalents

60 drops (gtt) = 1 teaspoon (t or tsp)
3 teaspoons (t or tsp) = 1 tablespoon (T or tbs)
2 tablespoons (T or tbs) = 1 ounce (f℥)

─────────── **10** ───────────

Now You Try It

Convert the following household equivalents using the ratio and proportion method.

a. f℥ II = _____ T

b. 3 tbs = _____ tsp

c. 13 tsp = _____ tbs

d. 45 gtt = _____ t

Units and Milliequivalents

─────────── **11** ───────────

You will notice two other measurements used to indicate a quantity of a prescribed medication: the unit (_____) and the milliequivalent (_____). Unit and milliequivalent quantities are measures that are independent of the metric, apothecary, and household systems of measurement.

known = want-to-know
gtt:tsp = gtt:tsp

$60:1 = x:\frac{2}{3}$

$60:1 = x:\frac{2}{3}$

$x = \dfrac{\overset{40}{\cancel{120}}}{\cancel{3}}$

$x = 40$ gtts

$\frac{2}{3}$ tsp = 40 gtts

a. f℥:T = f℥:T

$1:2 = 2:x$

$x = 4T$

b. t:T = t:T

$3:1 = x:3$

$x = 9t$

c. t:T = t:T

$3:1 = 13:x$

$\dfrac{\cancel{3}x}{\cancel{3}} = \dfrac{13}{3}$

$x = 4\frac{1}{3}t$

d. gtt:t = gtt:t

$60:1 = 45:x$

$\dfrac{\cancel{60}x}{\cancel{60}} = \dfrac{45}{60}$

$x = \frac{3}{4}t$

U

mEq

12
---

strength
potency

The unit (U) is a measure of the _____ or _____ of certain medications. Insulin, heparin, and penicillin are the medications most frequently dispensed in units. Just as the metric system and the apothecary system are unrelated, a unit of one medication **IS NOT THE SAME AMOUNT** as a unit of a different medication. For example, 1 U insulin is NOT the same amount as 1 U Heparin.

13
---

units

Dosages of insulin will be prescribed in _____, such as "35 U of Humulin N SQ @ 7:30 a.m."

14
---

heparin
penicillin

Two other medications frequently dispensed in units are _____ and _____.

15
---

potency/strength

Electrolytes are commonly prescribed in amounts of milliequivalents. Milliequivalents indicate the _____ or concentration of an electrolyte.

16
---

mEq

The electrolyte most frequently dispensed in milliequivalents is potassium chloride. You abbreviate milliequivalents as _____.

17

Now You Try It

Complete the following statements.

a. milliequivalents

a. Electrolytes may be prescribed in _____.

b. heparin,
   insulin, penicillin

b. Units are used to prescribe dosages of _____, _____, and _____.

c. mEq

c. The abbreviation for milliequivalent(s) is _____.

d. U

d. The abbreviation for unit(s) is _____.

⭐ What You've Achieved!

★ You know the basic units of the household system.

★ You always remember to express household volumes using correct notation and abbreviations.

★ You can define unit and milliequivalent.

★ You know how to convert household volumes from one unit of measure to another.

Great job! What you've learned in this chapter will help you calculate dosages prescribed in the household system. Before you move forward, take the review test to demonstrate your mastery of household measurements. If you get more than one wrong in any section, consider studying that portion of the chapter again.

Review Test

A

Complete the following statements.

1. The _____ and _____ systems of measurement are more accurate than the household system.

2. The three most common household measures used for self-administered medications are the _____, _____, and _____.

3. Dosages for penicillin, insulin, and heparin are usualy prescribed in _____.

4. Electrolytes, such as _____ _____, are often prescribed in milliequivalents.

B

Write the following measurements using correct notation rules and abbreviations.

5. twelve drops _____

6. twenty-five units _____

7. forty milliequivalents _____ **8.** nine tablespoons _____

9. seven teaspoons _____ **10.** four fluidounces _____

-- C --

Convert the following household equivalents using the ratio and proportion method.

11. 5 t = _____ T

12. f℥ V = _____ T

13. $\frac{2}{3}$ t= _____ gtts

14. 10 T = _____ t

15. 17 T = _____ f℥

16. 75 gtts = _____ t

17. 90 gtts = _____ T

18. 15 t = _____ f℥

Answers for Review Test

1. metric and apothecary   **2.** teaspoons, tablespoons, and drops   **3.** units

4. potassium chloride   **5.** 12 gtts   **6.** 25 U   **7.** 40 mEq

8. 9 T or 9 tbs   **9.** 7 t or 7 tsp   **10.** 4 f℥

---

11. t:T = t:T

$3:1 = 5:x$

$\frac{3x}{3} = \frac{5}{3}$

$x = 1\frac{2}{3}$ T

12. f℥:T = f℥:T

$1:2 = 5:x$

$x = 10$ T

13. t:gtt = t:gtt

$1:60 = \frac{2}{3}:x$

$x = \frac{\overset{20}{\cancel{60}}}{1} \times \frac{2}{\cancel{3}}$

$x = 40$ gtt

14. T:t = T:t

$1:3 = 10:x$

$x = 30$ t

---

15. T:f℥ = T:f℥

$2:1 = 17:x$

$\frac{2x}{2} = \frac{17}{2}$

$x = 8\frac{1}{2}$ f℥

16. gtt:t = gtt:t

$60:1 = 75:x$

$\frac{\cancel{60}x}{\cancel{60}} = \frac{75}{60}$

$x = 1\frac{1}{4}$ t

17. gtt:T = gtt:T

$180:1 = 90:x$

$\frac{\cancel{180}x}{\cancel{180}} = \frac{\cancel{90}}{\cancel{180}}$

$x = \frac{1}{2}$ T

18. t:f℥ = t:f℥

$6:1 = 15:x$

$\frac{\cancel{6}x}{\cancel{6}} = \frac{15}{6}$

$x = 2\frac{1}{2}$ f℥

Conversion Between Systems of Measurement

Objectives

When you finish this chapter, you will be able to:

★ State the common approximate liquid equivalents among the metric, apothecary, and household systems.

★ State the common approximate weight equivalents among the metric, apothecary, and household systems.

★ Convert units of weight and volume from one system of measurement to another.

Chapter Outline

★ Metric, Apothecary, and Household Equivalents

★ Converting Between Systems of Measurement

Introduction

You will use the metric system most frequently when administering medications and calculating drug dosages. On occasion, however, you will need to convert from one system of measurement to another. This need usually arises when a drug dosage is prescribed in one system and the available dosage is measured in another system. Converting a drug dosage from one system of measurement to another results in dosages that are **approximate equivalents** of each other, not exactly equal amounts. Further, because conversion tables vary in accuracy, you might calculate an equivalent dosage that varies as much as 10% from the original. Variations of 10% or less are acceptable in most cases, however.

Metric, Apothecary, and Household Equivalents

1

different

Conversion between one system of measurement and another is necessary when the prescribed dosage is written in a _____ system of measurement from the available dosage.

2

approximate

10%

The conversion result is an _____ equivalent of the same dosage in the original system of measurement. It may vary as much as _____ from the original measurement.

3

Table 8.1 lists approximate equivalencies you will use to convert between systems of measurement. You need only memorize six commonly used equivalents:

* 1 grain is equivalent to 60 milligrams,

* 15 grains is equivalent to 1 gram,

* 2.2 pounds is equivalent to 1 kilogram,

* 15 minims is equivalent to 1 milliliter,

* 1 fluidounce is equivalent to 30 milliliters,

* 1 teaspoon is equivalent to 5 milliliters.

equivalents

Remember, you can refer to the equivalency table for less frequently used _____.

TABLE 8.1 **Equivalency Table for Systems of Measurement**

	Volume	
Metric	*Apothecary*	*Household*
	1 minim (♏)	= 1 drop (gtt)
1 milliliter (mL)	= 15 or 16 minim (♏)	= 15 or 16 drops (gtt)
5 milliliters (mL)	= 1 fluidram (fʒ)	= 1 teaspoon (t)
15 milliliters (mL)	=	1 tablespoon (T)
30 milliliters (mL)	= 1 fluidounce (fʒ)	= 2 tablespoons (T)
500 milliliters (mL)	= 16 fluidounces (fʒ)	= 1 pint (pt)
1 liter (L) (1000 mL)	=	1 quart (qt)

Weights

Metric		Apothecary	Household
60 or 65 milligrams (mg)	=	1 grain (gr)	
1 gram (g) (1000 mg)	=	15 grains (gr)	
0.45 kilogram (kg)	=		1 pound (lb)
1 kilogram (kg) (1000 g)	=		2.2 pounds (lb)

──────────────── **4** ────────────────

Let's review. Fifteen minims is equivalent to _____ milliliter.

| | 1 |

──────────────── **5** ────────────────

Thirty milliliters is equivalent to _____ fluid-ounce.

| | 1 |

──────────────── **6** ────────────────

One teaspoon is equivalent to _____ milliliters.

| | 5 |

──────────────── **7** ────────────────

One kilogram is equivalent to _____ pounds.

| | 2.2 |

──────────────── **8** ────────────────

Fifteen grains is equivalent to _____ gram.

| | 1 |

──────────────── **9** ────────────────

And finally, one grain is equivalent to _____ milligrams.

| | 60 |

──────────────── **10** ────────────────

Look at Table 8.1. You will notice that one grain is equivalent to 60 *or* 65 milligrams. This is an example of the 10% or less variation allowance for conversion equivalencies. You will see both equivalents used by different pharmaceutical companies. For your calculations here, assume that 60 milligrams is equivalent to _____ grain.

| | 1 |

---------------------------------- **11** ----------------------------------

The equivalency table also indicates one milliliter is equivalent
to fifteen or sixteen minims. You will use the equivalency fifteen
minims is equal to _____ milliliter.

1

---------------------------------- **12** ----------------------------------

Again, let's look at Table 8.1. Although the table indicates one
minim is equivalent to _____ drop, it is more accurate
to use the equivalency given on the drug container because drops
vary in size with different drop dispensers.

1

>
> **REMEMBER**
> **Equivalent values indicate approximate amounts.**

---------------------------------- **13** ----------------------------------

Now You Try It

State the equivalent amount for each of the given measurements.

a. 1   **a.** 60 mg = gr _____

b. 15   **b.** 1 g   = gr _____

c. 2.2   **c.** 1 kg   = _____ lb

d. 15   **d.** 1 cc   = ℳ _____

e. 30   **e.** f℥ I   = _____ mL

f. 1   **f.** 5 cc   = _____ tsp

g. 15   **g.** 1 Tbs   = _____ cc

>
> **REMEMBER**
> **One milliliter (mL) is equal to one cubic centimeter (cc).**

Converting Between Systems of Measurement

—————————— **14** ——————————

Use the ratio-and-proportion method as outlined in Chapter 4 to convert between systems of measurement. To review, first select two equal ratios and write them as a proportion, labeled "known" ratio and "_____ _____ _____" ratio.

want-to-know

—————————— **15** ——————————

Next, write the units in proportional form and then write the _____ in proportional form.

quantities

—————————— **16** ——————————

Finally, multiply the means and extremes and solve for the _____ quantity.

unknown

—————————— **17** ——————————

For example, let's convert 45 minims of Robitussin to milliliters.

$$known = want\text{-}to\text{-}know$$

$$mL:\text{♏} = mL:\text{♏} \longleftarrow \text{units in proportional form}$$

$$1:15 = x:45 \longleftarrow \text{quantities in proportional form}$$

$$1:15 = x:45 \longleftarrow \text{multiply means and extremes}$$

$$15x = 45$$

$$\frac{\cancel{15}x}{\cancel{15}} = \frac{\cancel{45}^{3}}{\cancel{15}} \longleftarrow \text{cancel}$$

$$x = 3 \text{ mL}$$

Therefore, 45 minims is equivalent to 3 milliliters.

g:gr = g:gr

1:15 = 1.5:x

1:15 = 1.5:x

x = 22.5 gr

1.5 g = gr 22.5

gr:mg = gr:mg

1:60 = $\frac{1}{4}$:x

1:60 = $\frac{1}{4}$:x

$x = 60 \times \frac{1}{4}$

$x = 15$ mg

gr $\frac{1}{4}$ = 15 mg

a. mL:fʒ = mL:fʒ

30:1 = 320:x

$30x = 320$

$\frac{30x}{30} = \frac{320}{30}$

x = fʒ 10.7

b. ♏:cc = ♏:cc

15:1 = x:2.5

x = ♏ 37.5

c. gr:mg = gr:mg

1:60 = 10:x

$x = 600$ mg

18

Practice on this problem. Convert 1.5 grams of Robaxin to grains. _____

19

Convert morphine gr $\frac{1}{4}$ to milligrams. _____

20

Now You Try It

Convert the following measurements using the ratio-and-proportion method. Round your answers to the nearest tenth.

a. The patient drank 320 mL of juice. How many fluidounces is this? _____

b. The patient received 2.5 cc of gamma globulin. How many minims is this? _____

c. The physician ordered Aspirin gr X. How many milligrams is this? _____

d. A newborn weighs 7.5 lb. How many kilograms is this?

_____

d. lb:kg = lb:kg

$$2.2{:}1 = 7.5{:}x$$

$$2.2x = 7.5$$

$$\frac{2.2x}{2.2} = \frac{7.5}{2.2}$$

$$x = 3.4 \text{ kg}$$

☆ What You've Achieved!

★ You know the commonly used equivalents among the metric, apothecary, and household systems of measurement.

★ You always remember that conversions between metric, apothecary, and household systems of measurement result in approximate equivalents.

★ You can convert between different systems of measurement using the ratio and proportion method.

Fantastic! What you've learned in this chapter will help you calculate drug dosages when the prescribed dosage and available dosage are in different systems of measurement. Before moving forward, take the review test to demonstrate your mastery of converting between systems of measurement. If you get more than two wrong in either section, consider studying that portion of the chapter again.

Review Test

A

Convert the following measurements to the indicated units. Refer to the equivalency tables as needed. Round decimal answers to the nearest tenth.

1. gr Iss = _____ mg

2. ℥ 60 = _____ cc

3. 45 mL = _____ tsp

4. 35 t = _____ cc

5. 0.05 g = _____ mg

6. f℥ IIss = _____ cc

7. 12 mL = ℥ _____

8. 3 tbs = _____ mL

9. gr X = _____ g

10. 75 mL = _____ T

Solve the following word problems. Refer to the equivalency table as needed. Round decimal answers to the nearest tenth.

11. An infant drank ʒ $4\frac{2}{3}$. How many milliliters is this? _____

12. The physician orders 15 cc of Gelucil. How many teaspoons is this? _____

13. The physician orders "force fluids to 2750 mLs." How many liters is this? _____

14. A patient weighs 70 kg. How many pounds is this? _____

15. The physician orders morphine gr $\frac{1}{6}$. How many milligrams is this? _____

16. The patient drank 240 cc of juice. How many fluidounces is this? _____

17. The physician orders ASA gr V. How many milligrams is this? _____

18. The physician orders tetracycline 250 mg. How many grains is this? _____

19. A patient weighs 100 lb. How many kilograms is this? _____

20. The physician orders Provera 10 mg. How many grains is this? _____

Answers for Review Test

1. gr:mg = gr:mg

$$1:60 = 1.5:x$$

$$x = 90 \text{ mg}$$

2. cc:♏ = cc:♏

$$1:15 = x:60$$

$$15x = 60$$

$$\frac{15x}{15} = \frac{60}{15}$$

$$x = 4 \text{ cc}$$

3. mL:tsp = mL:tsp

$$5:1 = 45:x$$

$$5x = 45$$

$$\frac{5x}{5} = \frac{45}{5}$$

$$x = 9 \text{ tsp}$$

4. cc:tsp = cc:tsp

$$5:1 = x:35$$

$$x = 175 \text{ cc}$$

5. mg:g = mg:g

$$1000:1 = x:0.05$$

$$x = 50 \text{ mg}$$

6. fʒ:cc = fʒ:cc

$$1:30 = 2.5:x$$

$$x = 75 \text{ cc}$$

---

7. ℳ:mL = ℳ:mL

$$15:1 = x:12$$

$$x = ℳ180$$

8. mL:tbs = mL:tbs

$$15:1 = x:3$$

$$x = 45 \text{ mL}$$

9. g:gr = g:gr

$$1:15 = x:10$$

$$15x = 10$$

$$\frac{15x}{15} = \frac{10}{15}$$

$$x = 0.7 \text{ g}$$

---

10. T:mL = T:mL

$$1:15 = x:75$$

$$15x = 75$$

$$\frac{15x}{15} = \frac{75}{15}$$

$$x = 5 \text{ T}$$

11. mL:fʒ = mL:fʒ

$$30:1 = x:4\frac{2}{3}$$

$$x = \frac{\overset{10}{\cancel{30}}}{1} \times \frac{14}{\cancel{3}}$$

$$x = 140 \text{ mL}$$

12. tsp:cc = tsp:cc

$$1:5 = x:15$$

$$5x = 15$$

$$\frac{5x}{5} = \frac{15}{5}$$

$$x = 3 \text{ tsp}$$

---

13. L:mL = L:mL

$$1:1000 = x:2750$$

$$1000x = 2750$$

$$\frac{1000x}{1000} = \frac{2750}{1000}$$

$$x = 2.75 \text{ L}$$

$$x = 2.8 \text{ L}$$

14. kg:lb = kg:lb

$$1:2.2 = 70:x$$

$$x = 154 \text{ lb}$$

15. mg:gr = mg:gr

$$60:1 = x:\frac{1}{6}$$

$$x = \frac{\overset{10}{\cancel{60}}}{1} \times \frac{1}{\cancel{6}}$$

$$x = 10 \text{ mg}$$

---

16. f℥:c = f℥:cc

$1:30 = x:240$

$30x = 240$

$\dfrac{30x}{30} = \dfrac{240}{30}$

$x = $ f℥ VIII

17. mg:gr = mg:gr

$60:1 = x:5$

$x = 300$ mg

18. mg:gr = mg:gr

$60:1 = 250:x$

$60x = 250$

$\dfrac{60x}{60} = \dfrac{250}{60}$

$x = $ gr $4\dfrac{1}{6}$

19. kg:lb = kg:lb

$1:2.2 = x:100$

$2.2x = 100$

$\dfrac{2.2x}{2.2} = \dfrac{100}{2.2}$

$x = 45.45$ kg

$x = 45.5$ kg

20. gr:mg = gr:mg

$1:60 = x:10$

$60x = 10$

$\dfrac{60x}{60} = \dfrac{10}{60}$

$x = $ gr $\dfrac{1}{6}$

Dosage Preparation Skills

III

☆ When you need to administer a medication, the drug dosage ordered by the physician may be written in a different unit of measurement from that of the drug dosage on hand. In these situations, you will need to perform a dosage calculation in order to determine the exact quantity of medication to administer.

The ability to calculate dosages, however, is only one of the skills needed to accurately determine the quantity of medication to administer. You will also need to interpret medication labels and medication orders correctly, understand the use and calibrations of different syringes, and calculate oral and parenteral dosages. This section will help you master the skills necessary to safely and accurately prepare and administer medications.

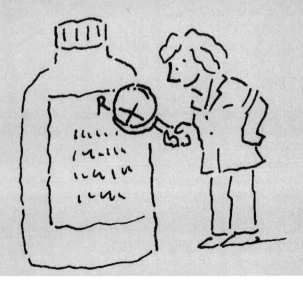

9

Reading Medication Labels and Orders

Objectives

When you finish this chapter, you will be able to:

★ Define and describe trade and generic drug names.

★ Identify the trade and generic names on medication labels.

★ Identify the preparation form, dosage strength, expiration date, and storage or preparation directions on a medication label.

★ Understand the importance of the expiration date on drug labels.

★ Identify and write common abbreviations in a medication order.

Chapter Outline

★ Reading Medication Labels

★ Expiration Dates

★ Reading Directions for Storing and Preparing Medications

★ Reading Medication Orders

Introduction

Medication Labels

All medications are labeled in a standard way according to federal standards. You will need to be able to interpret the information on medication labels in order to accurately prepare, administer, and store medications. Medication label information includes the drug's trade (brand) and generic (official) names, preparation form, dosage strength, and expiration date. You will also find directions for properly storing and preparing the drug. Sometimes not all of the information you need about a drug can be found on the medication label. In such cases, you must consult a pharmacist, the drug package insert, or one of a variety of drug references.

Medication Orders

The **medication order** is the format the physician uses to prescribe medication for the patient. The medication order includes the name of the drug, the dosage, the route of administration, and the frequency, or number of times the medication is to be administered. Abbreviations are frequently used to write the dosage, route, and frequency of administration of a medication order. You will need to interpret the medication order accurately before calculating the drug dosage and preparing the medication for administration.

Reading Medication Labels

1

A medication label lists the drug's _____ name (**brand name**) and _____ name (**official name**).

trade
generic

2

The **trade name**, or _____ name is chosen, copyrighted, and exclusively used by the pharmaceutical company that manufactures the drug. The first letter of the trade name is always capitalized. For example, Vistaril (Figure 9.1) is a trade name because the first letter is _____.

brand

capitalized

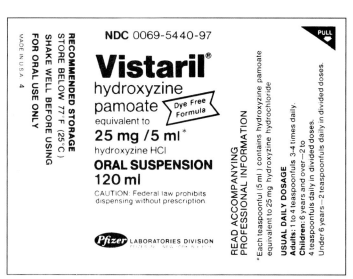

FIGURE 9.1

3

Sometimes the trade name is written in all capital letters. For example, Polycillin (Figure 9.2) is a trade name because _____ letters are capitalized.

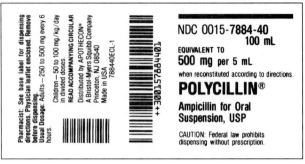

FIGURE 9.2

4

The trade name of a drug is followed by the symbol ® to the upper right of the name, indicating that the name is **registered**. For example, the symbol appearing to the right of Polycillin® (Figure 9.2) indicates that this is the drug's _____ trade name.

5

The drug's **generic**, or _____ name is derived from its chemical name. It is written in small or lowercase letters and is used regardless of which pharmaceutical company manufactured the drug. For example, hydroxyzine pamoate (Figure 9.1) is a generic name because all the letters are _____ .

6

The *United States Pharmacopeia* (**USP**) is an official drug reference. USP written after the generic name and preparation form on a drug label simply indicates that the drug is listed in the _____ _____ _____ . For example, in Figure 9.2, USP appears after Polycillin's generic name, ampicillin. You should be careful not to confuse USP with a drug name or preparation form.

all

registered

official

lowercase

*United States
Pharmacopeia*

---------------------- **7** ----------------------

A drug may have several trade names if it is manufactured by different pharmaceutical companies, but only _____ generic name. The physician may order the medication using the trade or generic name.

one

---------------------- **8** ----------------------

Look at the drug label for Cardizem (Figure 9.3). The trade name is _____, while the generic name is _____.

Cardizem
diltiazem HCl

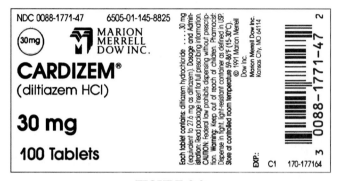

FIGURE 9.3

---------------------- **9** ----------------------

Drug manufacturers prepare medications in various **preparation forms**. A drug's preparation form is listed on the medication label. Drug preparation forms include tablets, capsules, oral suspensions, suppositories, lotions, ointments, and aqueous solutions. See Appendix B for examples of preparation forms. Looking again at Figure 9.3, we see that Cardizem is prepared in the form of _____, which is abbreviated "tab."

tablets

---------------------- **10** ----------------------

The **dosage strength** is the drug dose present in the preparation form. The dosage strength is always followed by a unit of measure, such as mg, g, gr, mEq, or U. In Figure 9.3, the dosage strength of Cardizem is _____.

30 mg/tablet

----------- **11** -----------

The dosage strength of a liquid includes the drug dose present in a volume of solution containing the dose. Don't confuse the drug dose with the total volume of solution. The volume amount is always followed by a unit of measure (such as mL, cc, ℥, f℥, tsp, or tbs). For example, in Figure 9.2, the dosage strength of Polycillin is _____.

500 mg/5 mL

>
>
> D I D Y O U N O T I C E ?
>
> **Most medication labels indicate the total quantity of medication in the drug container (such as 100 tablets, in Figure 9.3, and 100 mL, in Figure 9.2).**

----------- **12** -----------

Now You Try It

Record the following information from each medication label.

a. The label in Figure 9.4.

See package insert for complete product information.

Dispense in tight, light-resistant container.

Keep container tightly closed.

Store at controlled room temperature 15°-30° C (59°-86° F)

812 372 303

NDC 0009-0141-01
100 Tablets
6505-01-216-6289

Micronase®
Tablets
glyburide

2.5 mg

Caution: Federal law prohibits dispensing without prescription.

The Upjohn Company
Kalamazoo, MI 49001, USA

Upjohn

FIGURE 9.4

a. Micronase

   glyburide

   tablets

   2.5 mg/tablet

trade name _____

generic name _____

preparation form _____

dosage strength _____

b. The label in Figure 9.5.

See package insert for complete product information.

Dispense in tight, light-resistant container

Keep patient under close observation of a physician

Store at controlled room temperature 15°-30° C (59°-86° F)

810 338 203

The Upjohn Company
Kalamazoo, MI 49001 USA

NDC 0009-0049-02
100 Tablets

Medrol® 2 mg
Tablets

methylprednisolone
tablets, USP

Caution: Federal law prohibits dispensing without prescription.

Upjohn

FIGURE 9.5

trade name _____

generic name _____

preparation form _____

dosage strength _____

b. Medrol

methylprednisolone

tablets

2 mg/tablet

REMEMBER

Always write the quantity per unit when determining the dosage strength for solid preparation forms.

c. The label in Figure 9.6.

NDC 0009-0728-05
6505-01-246-8718
Not for direct infusion
Cleocin Phosphate®
Sterile Solution
clindamycin phosphate injection, USP
Equivalent to clindamycin
150 mg per ml
For intramuscular or intravenous use
Caution: Federal law prohibits dispensing without prescription.

Upjohn The Upjohn Company
Kalamazoo, MI 49001, USA

60 ml Pharmacy
Bulk Package

See package insert for complete product information.
Warning—If given intravenously, dilute before use.
Swab vial closure with an antiseptic solution. Dispense aliquots from the vial via a suitable dispensing device into infusion fluids under a laminar flow hood using aseptic technique. DISCARD VIAL WITHIN 24 HOURS AFTER INITIAL ENTRY.
Store at controlled room temperature 15°-30° C (59°-86° F)
Each ml contains: clindamycin phosphate equivalent to clindamycin 150 mg; also disodium edetate, 0.5 mg; benzyl alcohol 9.45 mg added as preservative. When necessary, pH was adjusted with sodium hydroxide and/or hydrochloric acid.
813 718 201   DATE/TIME ENTERED . . . .

150 mg per ml
Equivalent to clindamycin
clindamycin phosphate injection, USP
Cleocin Phosphate Sterile Solution

FIGURE 9.6

trade name _____

generic name _____

preparation form _____

dosage strength _____

c. Cleocin Phosphate

clindamycin phosphate solution

150 mg/mL

d. The label in Figure 9.7.

240 mL **NDC** 0081-0113-18

RETROVIR® Syrup
(ZIDOVUDINE)

Each 5 mL (1 teaspoonful) contains
zidovudine 50 mg and sodium benzoate 0.2% added as a preservative.

CAUTION: Federal law prohibits
dispensing without prescription.

U.S. Patent Nos. 4818538 (Product Patent);
4724232, 4833130, and 4837208 (Use Patents)

For indications, dosage, precautions, etc., see accompanying package insert.
Store at 15° to 25°C (59° to
77°F) and protect from light.

Made in U.S.A. 587016

BURROUGHS WELLCOME CO.
Research Triangle Park, NC 27709

LOT
EXP

FIGURE 9.7

d. Retrovir

   zidovudine

   syrup

   50 mg/5 mL

trade name _____

generic name _____

preparation form _____

dosage strength _____

DID YOU NOTICE?

**The generic name is located under the trade name and
frequently found in parentheses.**

Expiration Dates

13

The **expiration date** is a cutoff time after which the drug's pharmaceutical properties might change (such as lose their effectiveness). Medications should _____ be given after the expiration date on the medication label.

not

---------------- **14** ----------------

Expiration dates are abbreviated "exp." For example, in Figure 9.8, the expiration date for this unit of Zyloprim is _____.

1/94

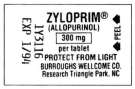

FIGURE 9.8

---------------- **15** ----------------

Medications that exceed their expiration date should be discarded on the last day of the month of the expiration date. For example, you should discard this unit of Zyloprim (Figure 9.8) on _____.

1/31/94

Reading Directions for Storing and Preparing Medications

---------------- **16** ----------------

You will find directions for storing and preparing medications on the medication labels. Read and follow these directions carefully to avoid errors. The next few frames will help you learn these skills.

---------------- **17** ----------------

Always read and follow any special directions regarding storage in order to maintain the potency and effectiveness of the medication. In the case of Cardizem (Figure 9.9, see page 108), the drug must be stored at a controlled room temperature of _____.

59°–86° F
(15°–30° C)

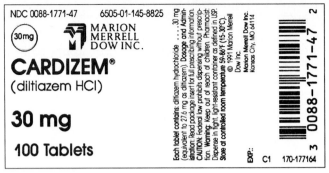

FIGURE 9.9

18

Now You Try It

Record the following information for each of the medication labels provided.

a. below 77° F
(below 25° C)

a. Ogen 5 (Figure 9.10) is stored at _____.

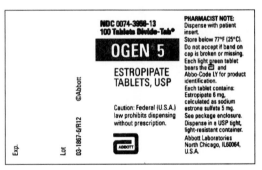

FIGURE 9.10

b. 59°–77° F
(15°–25° C)
light

b. Alkeran (Figure 9.11) is stored at _____ and protected from _____.

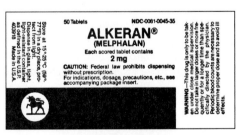

FIGURE 9.11

────────────── **19** ──────────────

Occasionally, a drug is packaged as a powder and must be reconstituted into a liquid before administration. Directions for the proper mixing or _____ of a drug are contained on the medication label.

reconstitution

────────────── **20** ──────────────

Read all directions for reconstitution carefully. If no directions are found on the medication label, read the drug package insert that accompanies the drug container. The drug package insert provides additional information about the medication not included on the medication label. Remember, you will read the _____ _____ _____ if reconstitution directions are not written on the medication label.

drug package insert

────────────── **21** ──────────────

After reading the directions, determine the amount of solution (called diluent or solvent) needed to reconstitute the medication. The reconstitution directions on the medication label for Ceclor (Figure 9.12) require that _____ of water be added to the drug container before use.

62 mL

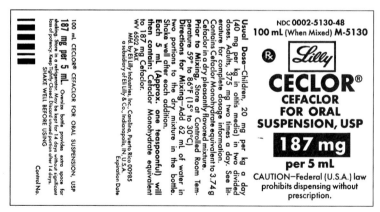

FIGURE 9.12

────────────── **22** ──────────────

In looking further at the directions for proper preparation of Ceclor (Figure 9.12), water must be added in _____ portions and _____ after each addition of water.

two
shaken well

187 mg/5 mL

14

a. oral suspension

   water

   47.6 mL

23

Next, determine the dosage strength after reconstitution. The dosage strength of Ceclor (Figure 9.12) is _____ .

REMEMBER

USP stands for *United States Pharmacopeia*, not a drug name or preparation form.

24

Finally, indicate the medication's expiration date by writing your initials and the date and time the medication was reconstituted on the medication label. For example, the expiration date of reconstituted Ceclor (Figure 9.12) is _____ days after reconstitution if the medication is refrigerated.

25

Now You Try It

Record the following information about each of the medication labels provided.

REMEMBER

To reconstitute a powdered medication:

Read the directions.
Determine the amount and type of the solvent.
Mix the powder and the solvent according to the directions on the medication label.
Determine the dosage strength of the liquid medication.
Indicate the expiration date by writing the date and time of reconstitution and your initials on the medication label.

a. Vibramycin label (Figure 9.13).

preparation form _____

type of diluent _____

amount of diluent _____

dosage strength _____   25 mg/5 mL

expiration instructions _____   Discard after 2 weeks

NDC 0069-0970-65

Vibramycin®

monohydrate

doxycycline monohydrate

FOR ORAL SUSPENSION

This package contains doxycycline monohydrate equivalent to **300 mg** of doxycycline in a raspberry-flavored mixture.†

60 ml BOTTLE

RASPBERRY FLAVORED

CAUTION: Federal law prohibits dispensing without prescription.

6277

Pfizer LABORATORIES DIVISION
PFIZER INC NEW YORK, N.Y. 10017

For oral use only

Mixing Directions: Tap bottle lightly to loosen powder. Add 47.6 ml of water to the bottle to make a total volume of 60 ml. Shake well.
When reconstituted, each teaspoonful (5 ml) contains doxycycline monohydrate equivalent to 25 mg of doxycycline.
doxycycline U.S. Pat. No. 3,200,149

RECOMMENDED STORAGE
STORE BELOW 86° F. (30° C.)
SHAKE WELL
This prescription, when in suspension, will maintain its potency for two weeks when kept at room temperature. Discard unused portion after two weeks.

MADE IN U.S.A. 9

READ ACCOMPANYING PROFESSIONAL INFORMATION
USUAL DOSAGE:
Adults: 200 mg on the first day (100 mg every 12 hours) followed by a maintenance dose of 100 mg a day.
Children above eight years of age: Under 100 lbs.— 2 mg/lb. of body weight daily divided in two doses on the first day, followed by 1 mg/lb. of body weight on subsequent days in one or two doses. Over 100 lbs.—See adult dosage.

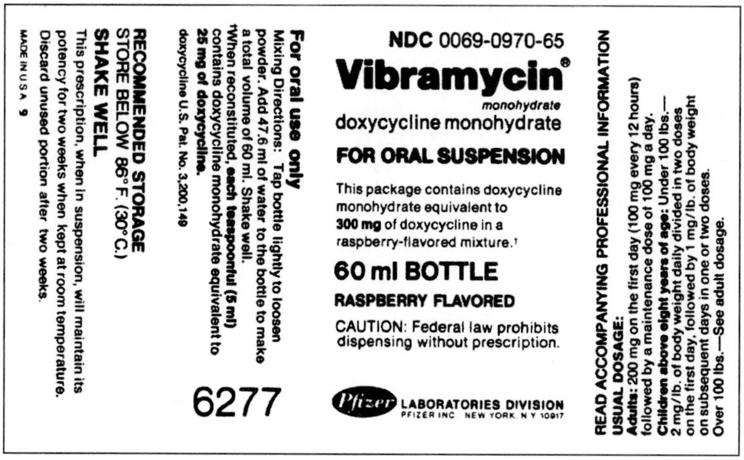

FIGURE 9.13

b. Cleocin Pediatric label (Figure 9.14).

preparation form _____   b. oral solution

type of diluent _____   water

amount of diluent _____   75 mL

dosage strength _____   75 mg/5 mL

expiration instructions _____   Discard after 2 weeks

NDC 0009-0760-04

Keep Container Tightly Closed

DO NOT REFRIGERATE SOLUTION

Store solution at room temperature

Shake well before each use

Discard any unused portion two weeks after reconstitution

Date of reconstitution _____

LOT

NDC 0009-0760-04   100 mL (when mixed)

Cleocin Pediatric®

Flavored Granules

clindamycin palmitate hydrochloride for oral solution, USP

75 mg per 5 mL

Equivalent to **75 mg per 5 mL** clindamycin when reconstituted

Upjohn Caution : Federal law prohibits dispensing without prescription.

Usual child dosage-5 mL (1 teaspoonful) four times daily.

See package insert for complete product information.

WARNING - NOT FOR INJECTION

Store unreconstituted product at controlled room temperature 15°-30° C (59°-86° F)
Reconstitute with a total of 75 mL of water as follows : add a large portion of the water and shake vigorously ; add remaining water and shake until solution is uniform. Each 5 mL (teaspoonful) of the solution contains clindamycin palmitate HCl equiv. to 75 mg clindamycin. Each bottle contains the equivalent of 1.5 grams clindamycin.

810 898 106   EXP

Made in Belgium for
The Upjohn Company
Kalamazoo, MI 49001, USA

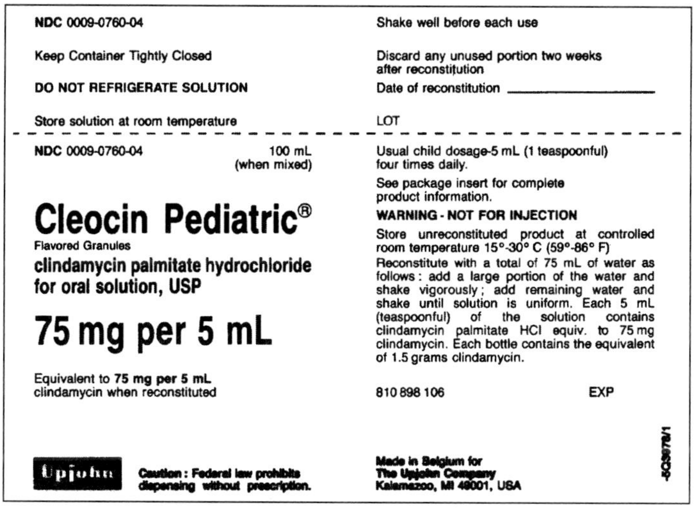

FIGURE 9.14

REMEMBER

Clarify all medication orders you don't understand by consulting a physician.

Reading Medication Orders

─────── **26** ───────

medication order

A _____ _____ includes the drug's name, dosage, and route and frequency of administration. You must understand the medication order perfectly before calculating the drug dosage and preparing the medication for administration.

─────── **27** ───────

route

The dosage, _____, and frequency of administration are abbreviated on the medication order. See Appendix A for a list of the most important abbreviations.

─────── **28** ───────

Let's examine a sample medication order:

Demerol 50 mg p.o. q.4h p.r.n. pain

milligrams

Referring to Appendix A, we can see that this order means: Demerol, 50 _____ , by mouth, every four hours, as needed for pain. Note that medication orders are usually written in the following order: drug, dosage, route, frequency. If any information is missing from a drug order, always consult a physician.

─────── **29** ───────

Now You Try It
Write in the meaning of the following abbreviations. Refer to Appendix A as needed.

a. The order reads: Seconal gr Iss p.o. h.s. p.r.n.

Written out: Seconal _____ (gr)

_____ (Iss) _____ (p.o.)

_____ (h.s.) _____ (p.r.n.)

b. The order reads: Septra 0.5 g p.o. t.i.d.

Written out: Septra 0.5 _____ (g)

_____ (p.o.) _____ (t.i.d.)

c. The order reads: Augmentin 250 mg p.o. q.6h.

Written out: Augmentin 250 _____ (mg)

_____ (p.o.) _____ (q.6h)

d. The order reads: K-Tab 10 mEq p.o. b.i.d.

Written out: K-Tab 10 _____ (mEq)

_____ p.o. _____ (b.i.d.)

a. grains
one and one half
by mouth
hour of sleep
as needed

b. gram
by mouth
three times a day

c. milligrams
by mouth
every six hours

d. milliequivalents
by mouth
twice a day

☆ What You've Achieved!

★ You know how to read the storage and preparation directions on medication labels.

★ You can differentiate between trade names and generic names.

★ You can determine the preparation form and dosage strength of drugs when reading a medication label.

★ You always remember to check the medication's expiration date.

★ You can identify and write common abbreviations used to prescribe medications.

Great job! What you've learned in this chapter will help you interpret medication labels and medication orders necessary for accurate preparation, administration, and storage of medications. Before moving forward, take the review test to demonstrate your mastery of reading medication orders and labels. If you get more than two wrong in section A or B, or one wrong in section C, consider studying that portion of the chapter again.

———————————————— **A** ————————————————

Indicate whether each statement characterizes a generic name (G) or a trade name (T) of a drug.

_____ **1.** It was selected and copyrighted by the pharmaceutical company producing the medication.

_____ **2.** It is usually written in small or lowercase letters.

_____ **3.** It is usually written with first letter capitalized or all letters capitalized.

_____ **4.** It is followed by the symbol ®.

_____ **5.** It is the same as the official name.

_____ **6.** It is derived from the chemical name.

_____ **7.** A drug may have only one of these names.

_____ **8.** It is also referred to as the brand name.

_____ **9.** A drug may have several of these types of names depending on the number of companies manufacturing the drug.

———————————————— **B** ————————————————

Record the following information about each of the medication labels provided.

10. The label in Figure 9.15:

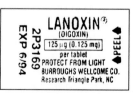

FIGURE 9.15

a. trade name _____

b. generic name _____

c. expiration date _____

11. The label in Figure 9.16:

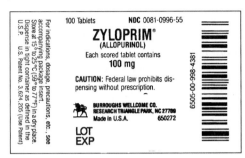

FIGURE 9.16

a. trade name _____

b. generic name _____

c. preparation form _____

d. dosage strength _____

12. The label in Figure 9.17:

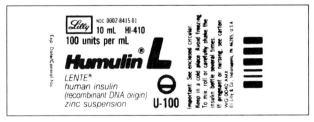

FIGURE 9.17

a. trade name _____

b. generic name _____

c. preparation form _____

d. dosage strength _____

13. The label in Figure 9.18:

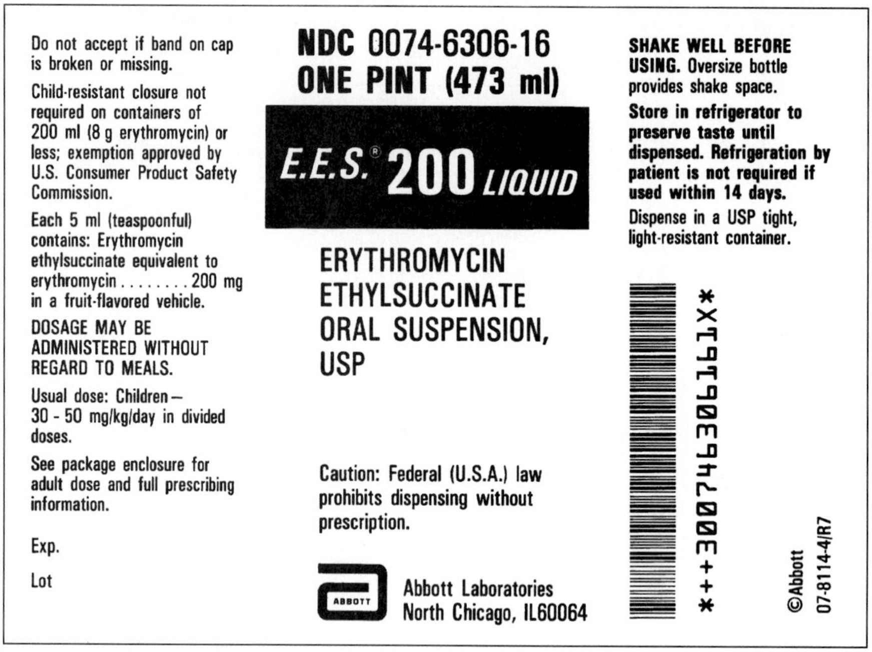

Do not accept if band on cap is broken or missing.

Child-resistant closure not required on containers of 200 ml (8 g erythromycin) or less; exemption approved by U.S. Consumer Product Safety Commission.

Each 5 ml (teaspoonful) contains: Erythromycin ethylsuccinate equivalent to erythromycin . . . . 200 mg in a fruit-flavored vehicle.

DOSAGE MAY BE ADMINISTERED WITHOUT REGARD TO MEALS.

Usual dose: Children— 30 - 50 mg/kg/day in divided doses.

See package enclosure for adult dose and full prescribing information.

Exp.

Lot

NDC 0074-6306-16
ONE PINT (473 ml)

E.E.S.® 200 LIQUID

ERYTHROMYCIN ETHYLSUCCINATE ORAL SUSPENSION, USP

Caution: Federal (U.S.A.) law prohibits dispensing without prescription.

Abbott Laboratories
North Chicago, IL60064

SHAKE WELL BEFORE USING. Oversize bottle provides shake space.

Store in refrigerator to preserve taste until dispensed. Refrigeration by patient is not required if used within 14 days.

Dispense in a USP tight, light-resistant container.

©Abbott
07-8114-4/R7

FIGURE 9.18

a. trade name _____

b. generic name _____

c. preparation form _____

d. dosage strength _____

14. The label in Figure 9.19:

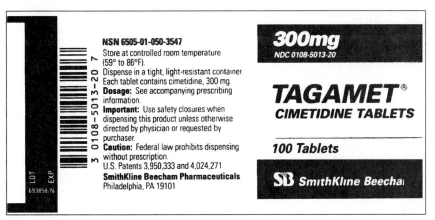

FIGURE 9.19

a. trade name _____

b. generic name _____

c. preparation form _____

d. dosage strength _____

15. The label in Figure 9.20:

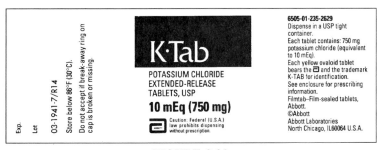

FIGURE 9.20

a. trade name _____

b. generic name _____

c. preparation form _____

d. dosage strength _____

16. The label in Figure 9.21:

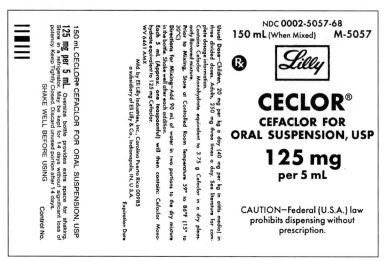

FIGURE 9.21

a. trade name _____

b. generic name _____

c. preparation form _____

d. amount of diluent _____

e. dosage strength _____

f. expiration instructions _____

17. The label in Figure 9.22:

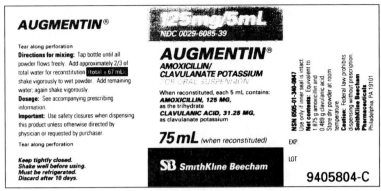

FIGURE 9.22

a. trade name _____

b. generic name _____

c. preparation form _____

d. amount of diluent _____

e. dosage strength _____

f. expiration instructions _____

---------------------------------- **C** ----------------------------------

Write out the meaning of the following abbreviations.

18. The order reads: ASA gr X p.o. q.4h. p.r.n. pain.

_____

19. The order reads: E.E.S. 0.5 g p.o. q.8h.

_____

20. The order reads: Tagamet 400 mg p.o. b.i.d. a.c.

_____

Answers for Review Test

1. T   2. G   3. T   4. T   5. G   6. G   7. G

8. T   9. T

---

10. a. Lanoxin
    b. digoxin
    c. 6/94

11. a. Zyloprim
    b. allopurinol
    c. tablets
    d. 100 mg/tab

12. a. Humulin L
    b. lente human insulin
    c. suspension
    d. 100 U/mL

---

13. a. E.E.S. 200 Liquid
    b. erythromycin ethylsuccinate
    c. oral suspension
    d. 200 mg/5mL

14. a. Tagamet
    b. cimetidine
    c. tablets
    d. 300 mg/tab

---

15. a. K-Tab
    b. potassium chloride
    c. extended-release tablets
    d. 10 mEq (750 mg)/tab

16. a. Ceclor
    b. cefaclor
    c. oral suspension
    d. 90 mL
    e. 125 mg/5 mL
    f. Discard after 14 days

---

17. a. Augmentin
    b. amoxicillin/clavulanate potassium
    c. oral suspension
    d. 67 mL
    e. Amoxicillin 125 mg and Clavulanic acid 31.25 mg/5 mL
    f. Discard after 10 days

---

18. ASA 10 grains by mouth every four hours as needed for pain.

---

19. E.E.S. 0.5 gram by mouth every eight hours.

---

20. Tagamet 400 milligrams by mouth twice a day before meals.

Oral Medications

Objectives

When you finish this chapter, you will be able to:

★ Name and explain the types of drug preparations used for oral administration.

★ Calculate dosages for oral medications in tablet, capsule, and liquid form.

Chapter Outline

★ Tablets, Capsules, and Liquids

★ Calculating Dosages of Tablets and Capsules

★ Dosages in Different Systems of Measurement

★ Calculating Liquid Dosages

Introduction

Medications are frequently administered by mouth. The oral route of administration is convenient and economical, and it is generally the safest for the patient. Usually oral medications are swallowed and then dissolved and absorbed by the upper gastrointestinal tract (the stomach and small intestine). These medications are available as solid and liquid preparations. Solid preparations include tablets and capsules. Orally administered liquid preparations include aqueous solutions, syrups, suspensions, and elixirs. A physician's medication order for an orally administered drug usually includes the drug name and dosage amount followed by the abbreviation "p.o." meaning *per os* (by mouth).

Tablets, Capsules, and Liquids

1

Oral medications are administered by _____.

mouth

Physicians usually order oral medications by using the abbreviation _____.

p.o.

Oral medications are available as _____ and _____ preparations.

solid
liquid

Orally administered liquid preparations may include _____, _____, _____, and _____.

syrups, elixirs,
aqueous solutions,
suspensions

_____ and _____ are two types of orally administered solid preparations.

Tablets
capsules

Pharmaceutical companies manufacture **tablets** in various sizes and forms. Many tablets are **scored**, as shown in Figure 10.1, so that they can be easily and accurately divided if a partial dosage is prescribed. Only _____ tablets should be broken.

scored

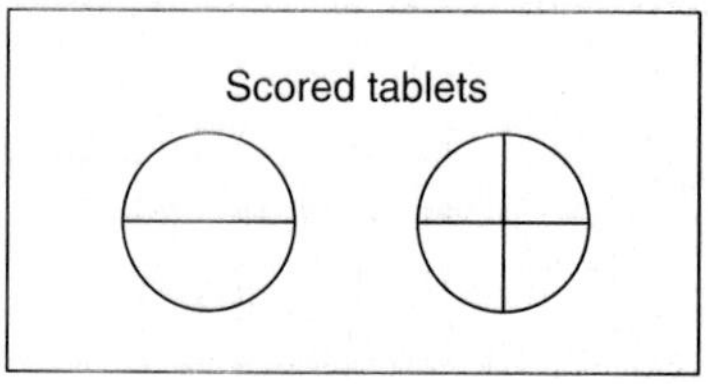

Scored tablets

FIGURE 10.1

Enteric-coated tablets have an outer coating that inhibits the tablet from dissolving in the stomach. It is important not to damage the coating. For this reason, enteric-coated tablets should not be broken, crushed or chewed. Enteric-coated tablets have a _____ _____.

special coating

--------- **8** ---------

Capsules are gelatin shells that may contain powders, liquids, or time-released granules. They should not be divided if a dose smaller than one capsule is required. Rather, a smaller capsule or a liquid preparation should be obtained from the pharmacist. Like an unscored or enteric-coated tablet, a _____ should be given as an entire unit.

capsule

Calculating Dosages of Tablets and Capsules

--------- **9** ---------

Frequently, the prescribed dosage of tablets and capsules is different from the _____ drug dosage.

available

 REMEMBER

Tablets and capsules are examples of solid preparation forms of medication.

--------- **10** ---------

Use the ratio-and-proportion method to calculate the number of tablets or capsules needed to administer the _____ dosage.

correct

--------- **11** ---------

Remember, the basic method involves three steps. First, select two equal ratios and write them as a proportion, labeled "known" ratio and " _____ _____ _____ " ratio. Second, write the units in proportional form and then write the quantities in proportional form. Third, multiply the means and the extremes and solve for the unknown quantity.

want-to-know

--------- **12** ---------

The available medication's dosage strength is used to determine the "known" ratio. Read the medication label to identify the _____ _____.

dosage strength

───────────────── **13** ─────────────────

The prescribed medication dosage is used to determine the "want-to-know" ratio. Read the medication order to determine the _____ dosage.

prescribed

───────────────── **14** ─────────────────

2 mg/tablet

Examine the label in Figure 10.2. The dosage strength for diazepam is _____. Let's determine the number of tablets to be administered for the order, "Diazepam 6 mg p.o."

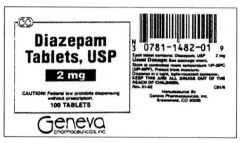

FIGURE 10.2

known ratio = want-to-know ratio

tab:mg = tab:mg ⟵ units in proportional form

$1:2 = x:6$ ⟵ quantities in proportional form

$1:2 = x:6$ ⟵ multiply means and extremes

$2x = 6$

$$\dfrac{2x}{2} = \dfrac{\overset{3}{\cancel{6}}}{\cancel{2}}$$ ⟵ cancel

$x = 3$ tablets

You will administer 3 tablets of Diazepam.

DID YOU NOTICE?

Diazepam is the generic name even though the first letter of the name is capitalized. Remember, official (generic) names listed in the *United States Pharmacopeia* are followed by the abbreviation USP.

───── **15** ─────

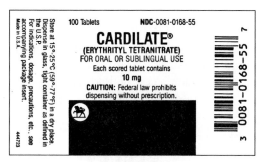

FIGURE 10.3

Look at the label in Figure 10.3. Calculate the number of tablets to administer for the order, "Cardilate 15 mg p.o. now." You will administer _____.

$$\text{tab:mg} = \text{tab:mg}$$
$$1:10 = x:15$$
$$1:10 = x:15$$
$$10x = 15$$
$$\frac{10x}{10} = \frac{15}{10}$$
$$x = 1.5$$

1.5 scored tablets of Cardilate

───── **16** ─────

Now You Try It

Calculate the following dosages using the ratio-and-proportion method.

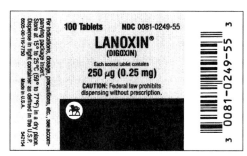

FIGURE 10.4

a. Examine the medication label in Figure 10.4. Determine the number of tablets you will administer for the order, "Lanoxin 0.125 mg p.o. q.d." You will administer _____.

a. $\text{tab:mg} = \text{tab:mg}$
$$1:0.25 = x:0.125$$
$$0.25x = 0.125$$
$$\frac{0.25x}{0.25} = \frac{0.125}{0.25}$$
$$x = 0.5 \text{ tab}$$

0.5 tabs of Lanoxin

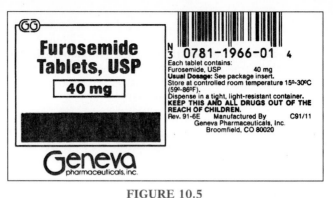

FIGURE 10.5

b. tab:mg = tab:mg

$1:40 = x:80$

$40x = 80$

$\dfrac{40x}{40} = \dfrac{80}{40}$

$x = 2$ tablets

2 tabs of furosemide

b. Examine the medication label in Figure 10.5. Determine the number of tablets you will administer for the order, "furosemide 80 mg p.o. b.i.d." You will administer _____.

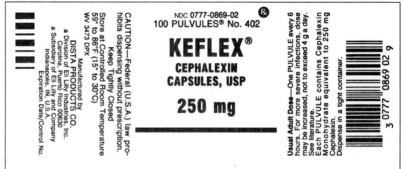

FIGURE 10.6

c. cap:mg = cap:mg

$1:250 = x:500$

$250x = 500$

$\dfrac{250x}{250} = \dfrac{500}{250}$

$x = 2$ capsules

2 caps of Keflex

c. Examine the medication label in Figure 10.6. Determine the number of capsules you will administer for the order, "Keflex 500 mg p.o. q.i.d." You will administer _____.

d. Determine the number of tablets you will administer for the order, "Synthroid 0.1 mg p.o. q.d." The available dosage is: Synthroid 0.05 mg/tab. You will administer _____.

d. tab:mg = tab:mg

$1:0.05 = x:0.1$

$0.05x = 0.1$

$\dfrac{0.05x}{0.05} = \dfrac{0.1}{0.05}$

$x = 2$ tablets

2 tabs of Synthroid

REMEMBER

Always check your answer by substituting the answer for the unknown quantity. The product of the means should equal the product of the extremes.

Dosages in Different Systems of Measurement

---- **17** ----

Occasionally, the prescribed dosage and the available drug dosage are in different units of measurement. To calculate the number of tablets or capsules to administer, the prescribed dosage and available dosage must be in the **same** units of measurement. To do this, you first convert the units of measurement to the _____ units and then solve the dosage problem.

same

---- **18** ----

FIGURE 10.7

Examine the label in Figure 10.7. Let's determine the number of tablets to administer for the order, "Aspirin gr X p.o. q.4h. p.r.n." First, convert the 10 grains to an equivalent number of milligrams. Use the ratio-and-proportion method, and refer to the equivalency tables found on the inside of the front and back covers.

known ratio = want-to-know ratio

gr:mg = gr:mg ⟵ **units in proportional form**

1:60 = 10:x ⟵ **quantities in proportional form**

1:60 = 10:x ⟵ **multiply means and extremes**

x = 600 mg

Therefore, gr X = _____ mg.

600

19

Once the prescribed amount of an order is in the same unit of measurement as the available drug dosage, determine the number of tablets to administer. Substitute 600 mg for gr X in the order.

known ratio = want-to-know ratio

tab:mg = tab:mg ⟵ units in proportional form

$1:325 = x:600$ ⟵ quantities in proportional form

$1:325 = x:600$ ⟵ multiply means and extremes

$325x = 600$

$$\frac{325x}{325} = \frac{600}{325}$$ ⟵ cancel

aspirin

$x = 1.846$ tablets of _____.

REMEMBER

The equivalency table values yield approximate amounts.

20

Remember, tablets can only be given as whole or half tablets, so in calculating dosage round to the nearest whole number (or half number, if scored).

2 tablets

Therefore, you will administer _____ _____ of aspirin. In situations where dosage is critical, the physician or pharmacist will clarify the dosage.

DID YOU NOTICE?

If 65 mg were used from the equivalency table instead of 60 mg, gr X would equal 650 mg, and the answer would yield exactly 2 tablets.

21

Now You Try It

Calculate the following dosages using the ratio-and-proportion method.

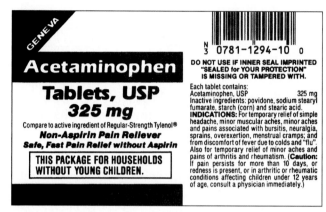

FIGURE 10.8

a. Examine the medication label in Figure 10.8. Determine the number of tablets you will administer for the order, "acetaminophen gr XV p.o. q.4–6h p.r.n., not to exceed 4 times/day." You will administer _____.

a. mg:gr = mg:gr
  60:1 = x:15

  60:1 = x:15

  $x = 900$ mg

  tab:mg = tab:mg
  1:325 = x:900

  1:325 = x:900

  $\dfrac{325x}{325} = \dfrac{900}{325}$

  $x = 2.77$ tablets
  $x = 3$ tablets

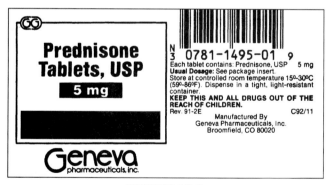

FIGURE 10.9

b. Examine the medication label in Figure 10.9. Determine the number of tablets you will administer for the order, "prednisone gr $\frac{1}{4}$ p.o. now." You will administer _____.

b. mg:gr = mg:gr
  $60:1 = x:\dfrac{1}{4}$

  $60:1 = x:\dfrac{1}{4}$

  $\qquad\quad 15$
  $x = \dfrac{\cancel{60}}{1} \times \dfrac{1}{\cancel{4}}$

  $x = 15$ mg

  tab:mg = tab:mg
  1:5 = x:15

  1:5 = x:15

  $\dfrac{\cancel{5}x}{\cancel{5}} = \dfrac{15}{5}$

  $x = 3$ tablets

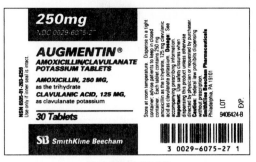

FIGURE 10.10

c. g:mg = g:mg
$$1:1000 = 0.5:x$$
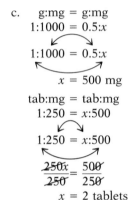
$$1:1000 = 0.5:x$$

$$x = 500 \text{ mg}$$

tab:mg = tab:mg
$$1:250 = x:500$$

$$1:250 = x:500$$

$$\frac{250x}{250} = \frac{500}{250}$$

$$x = 2 \text{ tablets}$$

c. Examine the medication label in Figure 10.10. Determine the number of tablets you will administer for the order, "Augmentin 0.5 g p.o. q.8h." You will administer _____.

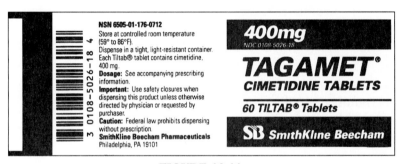

FIGURE 10.11

d. g:mg = g:mg
$$1:1000 = 0.8:x$$

$$1:1000 = 0.8:x$$

$$x = 800 \text{ mg}$$

tab:mg = tab:mg
$$1:400 = x:800$$

$$1:400 = x:800$$

$$\frac{400x}{400} = \frac{800}{400}$$

$$x = 2 \text{ tablets}$$

d. Examine the medication label in Figure 10.11. Determine the number of tablets you will administer for the order, "Tagament 0.8 g p.o. h.s." You will administer _____.

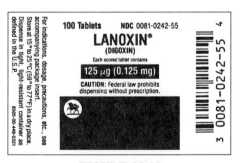

FIGURE 10.12

e. Examine the medication label in Figure 10.12. Determine the number of tablets you will administer for the order, "digoxin 0.25 mg p.o. q.d." You will administer _____.

> **REMEMBER**
>
> Always recheck calculations that seem unlikely (unusually large or small). Always have someone check your computations if you are uncertain about your calculations.

Calculating Liquid Dosages

22

Liquid preparations include aqueous solutions, syrups, suspensions, and elixirs. The drug dosage is contained within a specific volume, such as mL, cc, f℥, tsp, and tbs. The dosage strength of a liquid therefore includes the drug dosage per _____ of solution containing the dose. Dosage calculations for liquids follow the same procedure as for tablets.

volume

23

Let's review the three steps. First, select the two equal ratios and write them as a proportion, labeled the "known" ratio and the "want-to-know" ratio. The dosage strength becomes the "_____" ratio and the _____ _____ becomes the "want-to-know" ratio. Second, write the units in proportional form and then write the quantities in proportional form. Third, multiply the means and the extremes and solve for the unknown quantity.

known
prescribed dosage

24

Look at the medication label in Figure 10.13 (see page 132). Let's determine the volume of medication you will administer for the order, "Keflex suspension 200 mg p.o. q.i.d."

known ratio = want-to-know ratio

mg:mL = mg:mL ⟵ units in proportional form

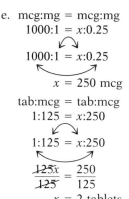

e. mcg:mg = mcg:mg
1000:1 = x:0.25

1000:1 = x:0.25

x = 250 mcg

tab:mcg = tab:mcg
1:125 = x:250

1:125 = x:250

$$\frac{\cancel{125}x}{\cancel{125}} = \frac{250}{125}$$

x = 2 tablets

$$125:5 = 200:x \quad \longleftarrow \text{quantities in proportional form}$$

$$125:5 = 200:x \quad \longleftarrow \text{multiply means and extremes}$$

$$\frac{\cancel{125}x}{\cancel{125}} = \frac{1000}{125} \quad \longleftarrow \text{cancel}$$

$$x = 8 \text{ mL}$$

8 mL

Therefore, you will administer _____ of Keflex suspension.

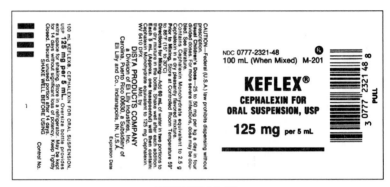

FIGURE 10.13

— **25** —

Now You Try It
Calculate the following dosages.

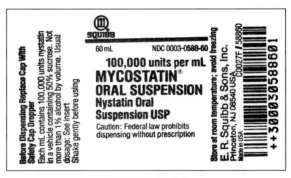

FIGURE 10.14

a. U:mL = U:mL
100000:1 = 250000:x

100000:1 = 250000:x

$$\frac{100000x}{100000} = \frac{250000}{100000}$$

x = 2.5 mL
nystatin

a. Examine the label in Figure 10.14. Determine the volume of medication you will administer for the order, "nystatin 250,000 U p.o. q.i.d." You will administer _____.

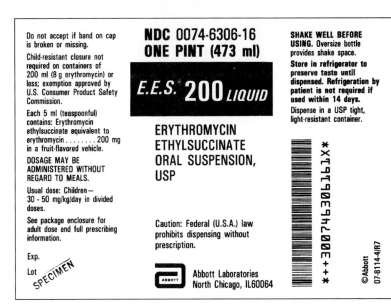

FIGURE 10.15

b. Examine the label in Figure 10.15. Determine the volume of medication you will administer for the order, "E.E.S. 160 mg p.o. q.6h." You will administer _____.

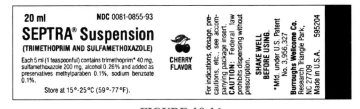

FIGURE 10.16

c. Examine the label in Figure 10.16. Determine the volume of medication you will administer for the order, "Sulfamethoxazole 0.35 g p.o. t.i.d." You will administer _____.

 REMEMBER
Use the equivalency tables found on the inside of the front and back covers.

d. The available dosage is: Benadryl 12.5 mg/5 cc. Determine the volume of medication you will administer for the order, "Benadryl elixir 25 mg p.o. now." You will administer _____.

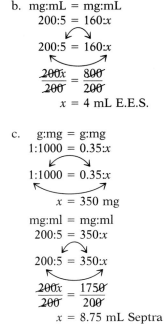

b. mg:mL = mg:mL
200:5 = 160:x

200:5 = 160:x

$\dfrac{200x}{200} = \dfrac{800}{200}$

x = 4 mL E.E.S.

c. g:mg = g:mg
1:1000 = 0.35:x

1:1000 = 0.35:x

x = 350 mg

mg:ml = mg:ml
200:5 = 350:x

200:5 = 350:x

$\dfrac{200x}{200} = \dfrac{1750}{200}$

x = 8.75 mL Septra

d. mg:cc = mg:cc
12.5:5 = 25:x

12.5:5 = 25:x

$\dfrac{12.5x}{12.5} = \dfrac{125}{12.5}$

x = 10 cc Benadryl

⭐ What You've Achieved!

★ You know how to convert the prescribed dosage and available dosage to the same unit of measurement before calculating dosages.

★ You know how to calculate dosages for oral medications in tablet, capsule, and liquid form.

★ You always remember to check your answers for accuracy.

Fantastic! What you've learned in this chapter will help you calculate dosages for oral medications. Before moving forward, take the review test to demonstrate your mastery of tablet, capsule, and oral liquid dosage calculations. If you get more than one wrong in any section, consider reading that portion of the chapter again.

Review Test

A

Determine the number of tablets you will administer for each problem using the medication labels provided.

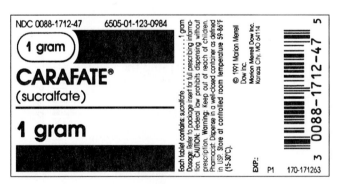

FIGURE 10.17

1. Look at Figure 10.17. The drug order reads: Carafate 500 mg p.o. b.i.d. You will administer _____.

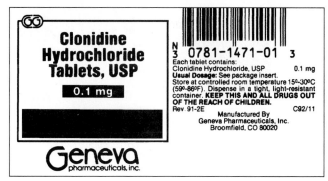

FIGURE 10.18

2. Look at Figure 10.18. The drug order reads: clonidine 0.3 mg p.o. q.d. You will administer _____.

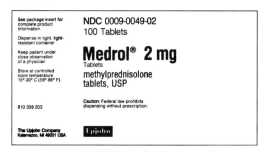

FIGURE 10.19

3. Look at Figure 10.19. The drug order reads: Medrol 8 mg p.o. q.d. You will administer _____.

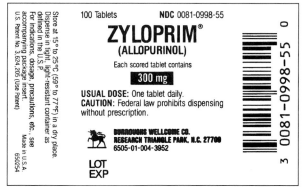

FIGURE 10.20

4. Look at Figure 10.20. The drug order reads: allopurinol 150 mg p.o. b.i.d. You will administer _____.

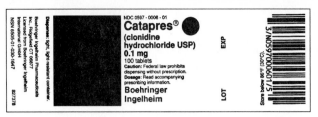

FIGURE 10.21

5. Look at Figure 10.21. The drug order reads: Catapres 300 mcg p.o. b.i.d. You will administer _____.

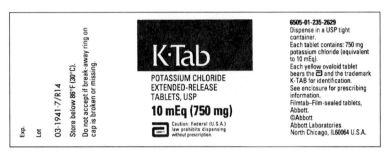

FIGURE 10.22

6. Look at Figure 10.22. The drug order reads: K-Tab 20 mEq p.o. b.i.d. You will administer _____.

B

Determine the number of tablets you will administer for each problem using the given available dosage.

7. The available dosage is: Verapamil 40 mg/tablet. The drug order reads: Verapamil 120 mg p.o. b.i.d. You will administer _____.

8. The available dosage is: thyroid 30 mg/tab. The drug order reads: thyroid gr I p.o. q.d. You will administer _____.

9. The available dosage is: Seconal 100 mg/capsule. The drug order reads: Seconal gr Iss p.o. h.s. p.r.n. You will administer _____.

10. The available dosage is: Synthroid 50 mcg/tablet. The drug order reads: Synthroid 0.15 mg p.o. q.d. You will administer _____.

—————————————————— **c** ——————————————————

Determine the volume of medication you will administer for each problem using the medication label provided.

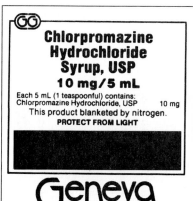

Chlorpromazine Hydrochloride Syrup, USP
10 mg/5 mL

Each 5 mL (1 teaspoonful) contains:
Chlorpromazine Hydrochloride, USP   10 mg
This product blanketed by nitrogen.
PROTECT FROM LIGHT

Geneva pharmaceuticals, inc.

N 3   0781-4017-04   1

Usual Dosage: See package insert.
Caution: Avoid direct contact with skin or clothes because of possibility of contact dermatitis (skin reaction). Wash thoroughly or change clothes if direct contact occurs.
Store at controlled room temperature 15º-30ºC (59º-86ºF).
Important: Dispense only in a tight **amber glass** container. This product is light sensitive. Never dispense in a flint, green, or blue bottle.
KEEP THIS AND ALL DRUGS OUT OF THE REACH OF CHILDREN.
Rev. 92-1E   C92/7

Manufactured By
Geneva Pharmaceuticals, Inc.
Broomfield, CO 80020

FIGURE 10.23

11. Look at Figure 10.23. The order reads: chlorpromazine 25 mg p.o. q.i.d. You will administer _____.

240 mL   NDC 0081-0113-18

RETROVIR® Syrup
(ZIDOVUDINE)

Each 5 mL (1 teaspoonful) contains zidovudine 50 mg and sodium benzoate 0.2% added as a preservative.

CAUTION: Federal law prohibits dispensing without prescription.

U.S. Patent Nos. 4818538 (Product Patent); 4724232, 4833130, and 4837208 (Use Patents)

For indications, dosage, precautions, etc., see accompanying package insert.
Store at 15° to 25°C (59° to 77°F) and protect from light.
Made in U.S.A.   587016

BURROUGHS WELLCOME CO.
Research Triangle Park, NC 27709

LOT
EXP

FIGURE 10.24

12. Look at Figure 10.24 (see page 137). The order reads: zidovudine 180 mg p.o. q.4h. You will administer _____.

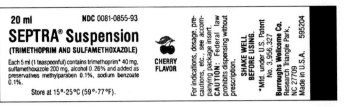

FIGURE 10.25

13. Look at Figure 10.25. The order reads: sulfamethoxazole 0.5 g p.o. t.i.d. You will administer _____.

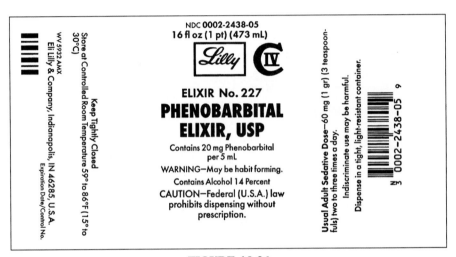

FIGURE 10.26

14. Look at Figure 10.26. The order reads: phenobarbitol elixir 50 mg p.o. t.i.d. You will administer _____.

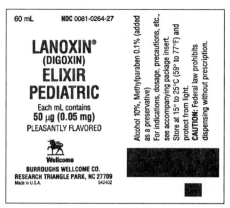

FIGURE 10.27

15. Look at Figure 10.27. The order reads: Lanoxin 0.15 mg p.o. q.d. You will administer _____.

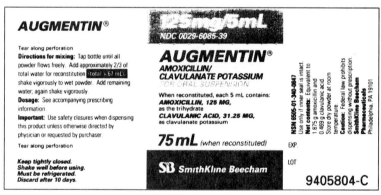

FIGURE 10.28

16. Look at Figure 10.28. The order reads: amoxicillin 0.175 g p.o. q.8h. You will administer _____.

Determine the volume of medication you will administer using the given available dosage.

17. The available dosage is: ampicillin 250 mg/5 cc. The order reads: ampicillin 0.4 g p.o. q.i.d. You will administer _____.

18. The available dosage is: guaifenesen 100 mg/1 cc. The order reads: guaifenesen syrup 0.25 g p.o. p.r.n. You will administer _____.

19. The available dosage is: KCl Elixir 20 mEq/15 cc. The order reads: KCl Elixir 15 mEq p.o. b.i.d. You will administer _____.

20. The available dosage is: acetaminophen 160 mg/5 cc. The order reads: acetaminophen elixir 240 mg p.o. q.4hr p.r.n. You will administer _____.

Answers for Review Test

1. mg:tab = mg:tab

$$1000:1 = 500:x$$

$$\frac{1000x}{1000} = \frac{500}{1000}$$

$$x = 0.5 \text{ tab}$$

0.5 tablets of Carafate

2. mg:tab = mg:tab

$$0.1:1 = 0.3:x$$

$$\frac{0.1x}{0.1} = \frac{0.3}{0.1}$$

$$x = 3 \text{ tabs}$$

3 tablets of clonidine

3. mg:tab = mg:tab

$$2:1 = 8:x$$

$$\frac{2x}{2} = \frac{8}{2}$$

$$x = 4 \text{ tabs}$$

4 tablets of Medrol

4. mg:tab = mg:tab

$$300:1 = 150:x$$

$$\frac{300x}{300} = \frac{150}{300}$$

$$x = 0.5 \text{ tabs}$$

0.5 tablets of Zyloprim

5. mg:mcg = mg:mcg

$$1:1000 = 0.1:x$$

$$x = 100 \text{ mcg}$$

mcg:tab = mcg:tab

$$100:1 = 300:x$$

$$\frac{100x}{100} = \frac{300}{100}$$

$$x = 3 \text{ tabs}$$

3 tablets of Catapres

6. mEq:tab = mEq:tab

$$10:1 = 20:x$$

$$\frac{10x}{10} = \frac{20}{10}$$

$$x = 2 \text{ tabs}$$

2 tablets of K-Tab

7. mg:tab = mg:tab

$40:1 = 120:x$

$$\frac{40x}{40} = \frac{120}{40}$$

$x = 3$ tabs

3 tablets of Verapamil

8. 60 mg = gr I

mg:tab = mg:tab

$30:1 = 60:x$

$$\frac{30x}{30} = \frac{60}{30}$$

$x = 2$ tabs

2 tablets of thyroid

9. gr:mg = gr:mg

$1:60 = 1.5:x$

$x = 90$ mg

mg:cap = mg:cap

$100:1 = 90:x$

$$\frac{100x}{100} = \frac{90}{100}$$

$x = 0.9 = 1$ cap

1 capsule of Seconal

---

10. mg:mcg = mg:mcg

$1:1000 = 0.15:x$

$x = 150$ mcg

mcg:tab = mcg:tab

$50:1 = 150:x$

$$\frac{50x}{50} = \frac{150}{50}$$

$x = 3$ tabs

3 tablets of Synthroid

11. mg:mL = mg:mL

$10:5 = 25:x$

$$\frac{10x}{10} = \frac{125}{10}$$

$x = 12.5$ mL

12.5 mL chlorpromazine hydrochloride

---

12. mg:mL = mg:mL

$50:5 = 180:x$

$$\frac{50x}{50} = \frac{900}{50}$$

$x = 18$ mL

18 mL Retrovir

13. g:mg = g:mg

$1:1000 = 0.5:x$

$x = 500$ mg

mg:mL = mg:mL

$200:5 = 500:x$

$$\frac{200x}{200} = \frac{2500}{200}$$

$x = 12.5$ mL

12.5 mL Septra

14. mg:mL = mg:mL

$$20:5 = 50:x$$

$$\frac{20x}{20} = \frac{250}{20}$$

$$x = 12.5 \text{ mL}$$

12.5 mL phenobarbitol elixir

15. mg:mL = mg:mL

$$0.05:1 = 0.15:x$$

$$\frac{0.05x}{0.05} = \frac{0.15}{0.05}$$

$$x = 3 \text{ mL}$$

3 mL Lanoxin Elixir

---

16. g:mg = g:mg

$$1:1000 = 0.175:x$$

$$x = 175 \text{ mg}$$

mg:mL = mg:mL

$$125:5 = 175:x$$

$$\frac{125x}{125} = \frac{875}{125}$$

$$x = 7 \text{ mL}$$

7 mL Augmentin

17. g:mg = g:mg

$$1:1000 = 0.4:x$$

$$x = 400 \text{ mg}$$

mg:cc = mg:cc

$$250:5 = 400:x$$

$$\frac{250x}{250} = \frac{2000}{250}$$

$$x = 8 \text{ cc}$$

8 cc ampicillin

18. g:mg = g:mg

$$1:1000 = 0.25:x$$

$$x = 250 \text{ mg}$$

mg:cc = mg:cc

$$100:1 = 250:x$$

$$\frac{100x}{100} = \frac{250}{100}$$

$$x = 2.5 \text{ cc}$$

2.5 cc guaifenesen

---

19. mEq:cc = mEq:cc

$$20:15 = 15:x$$

$$\frac{20x}{20} = \frac{225}{20}$$

$$x = 11.25 \text{ cc}$$

11.25 cc KCl Elixir

20. mg:cc = mg:cc

$$160:5 = 240:x$$

$$\frac{160x}{160} = \frac{1200}{160}$$

$$x = 7.5 \text{ cc}$$

7.5 cc acetaminophen elixir

Parenteral Medications

Objectives

When you finish this chapter, you will be able to:

★ Calculate the dosages for injectable medications dispensed from ampules and vials.

★ Follow the directions on drug labels or package inserts to reconstitute drugs packaged in powdered forms and to determine dosage strength.

★ Calculate the dosages for injectable medications requiring reconstitution.

Chapter Outline

★ Types and Characteristics of Parenteral Medications

★ Calculating Parenteral Medications

★ Reconstituting Powdered Parenteral Drugs

Introduction

Injection Types

Parenteral medications are sterile drug solutions administered by injection, using a sterile needle and syringe. Injections are given intramuscularly (IM, in a muscle), subcutaneously (SQ or SC, in adipose tissue), or intravenously (IV, in a vein). The average volume of drug administered SQ is 1 cc or less per site and 1–3 cc for IM in a single dose.

Package Forms

Injectable medications are packaged in ampules (single-use glass containers), single or multidose vials (rubber-stoppered glass containers), or prefilled cartridges (syringes prefilled with medication ready to use). Injectable medications are also packaged as a liquid or in a powdered form that requires reconstitution. Because the medication must be administered as a solution, the unit of measurement used with parenteral medications is always mL, cc, or ℥.

Types and Characteristics of Parenteral Medications

1

injection

Parenteral medications are those administered by _____.

2

sterile

Medications administered by injection require drug solutions that are _____. This required sterile preparation is noted on the drug label, and indicates the drug is suitable to administer parenterally.

3

intramuscular

The common parenteral routes are intravenous, subcutaneous, and _____.

4

intramuscularly (IM)
intravenously (IV)

Information regarding the specific route a medication can be administered is usually on the drug label. Cleocin (Figure 11.1) can be administered _____ or _____. (Note the term "sterile solution" under the trade name.)

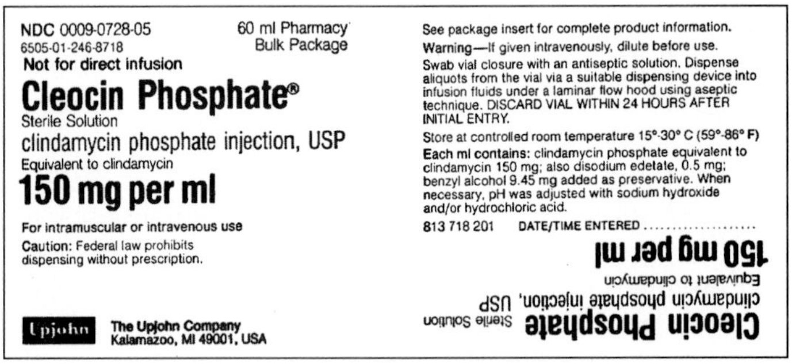

NDC 0009-0728-05   60 ml Pharmacy
6505-01-246-8718   Bulk Package
Not for direct infusion

Cleocin Phosphate®
Sterile Solution
clindamycin phosphate injection, USP
Equivalent to clindamycin

150 mg per ml

For intramuscular or intravenous use
Caution: Federal law prohibits
dispensing without prescription.

Upjohn The Upjohn Company
             Kalamazoo, MI 49001, USA

See package insert for complete product information.
Warning—If given intravenously, dilute before use.
Swab vial closure with an antiseptic solution. Dispense
aliquots from the vial via a suitable dispensing device into
infusion fluids under a laminar flow hood using aseptic
technique. DISCARD VIAL WITHIN 24 HOURS AFTER
INITIAL ENTRY.
Store at controlled room temperature 15°-30° C (59°-86° F)
Each ml contains: clindamycin phosphate equivalent to
clindamycin 150 mg; also disodium edetate, 0.5 mg;
benzyl alcohol 9.45 mg added as preservative. When
necessary, pH was adjusted with sodium hydroxide
and/or hydrochloric acid.
813 718 201   DATE/TIME ENTERED . . . .

150 mg per ml
Equivalent to clindamycin
clindamycin phosphate injection, USP
Cleocin Phosphate Sterile Solution

FIGURE 11.1

---------------------------------- **5** ----------------------------------

Intramuscular injections, abbreviated _____, are given into a _____.

| IM |
| muscle |

---------------------------------- **6** ----------------------------------

Subcutaneous injections, abbreviated _____ or _____ are given into _____ or fatty tissue.

| SQ |
| SC |
| adipose |

---------------------------------- **7** ----------------------------------

When a medication is injected into a vein, it is given _____, which is abbreviated _____.

| intravenously |
| IV |

---------------------------------- **8** ----------------------------------

Dosage strength for injections is the drug dose present in the _____ of solution. The volume amount is designated by a unit of measure such as mL, cc, or ℳ.

| volume |

---------------------------------- **9** ----------------------------------

The drug dosage within the solution is indicated by measurements such as mcg, mg, g, gr, U, and mEq. For instance, the dosage strength for Cleocin in Figure 11.1 is _____.

| 150 mg/mL |

---------------------------------- **10** ----------------------------------

It is important to check the labels on vials, ampules, and prefilled cartridges for expiration dates. If the expiration date has been exceeded, the medication should be _____.

| discarded |

> REMEMBER
>
> Labels of most parenteral medications are very small and must be read with particular care.

---------------------------------- **11** ----------------------------------

Now You Try It

Determine the dosage strength for each of the following medications using the medication labels provided.

80 mg/mL

a. Look at Figure 11.2. The dosage strength is _____.

FIGURE 11.2

0.4 mg/mL

b. Look at Figure 11.3. The dosage strength is _____.

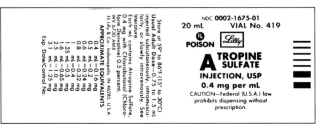

FIGURE 11.3

10,000 U/mL

c. Look at Figure 11.4. The dosage strength is _____.

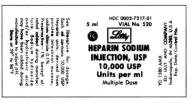

FIGURE 11.4

125 mg/mL
(1 g/8 mL)

d. Look at Figure 11.5. The dosage strength is _____.

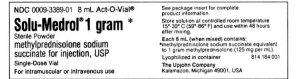

FIGURE 11.5

DID YOU NOTICE?

The parenteral drug containers indicate the total volume contained in each ampule or vial. For example, in Figure 11.2, Depo-Medrol's container holds 5 mL of medication.

Calculating Parenteral Medications

---- **12** ----

When the drug dosage available is identical to the physician's order, you do not have to calculate the drug dosage. The liquid amount containing the prescribed amount of medication is injected in its entirety. For example, look at Figure 11.6. If the physician orders "Dolophine 10 mg IM for pain" only _____ mL would be given.

one

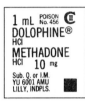

FIGURE 11.6

---- **13** ----

Ampules and prefilled cartridges contain 0.1 to 0.2 mL excess drug in case of accidental drug loss while preparing the medication for injection. You must not assume that the prescribed dosage is the entire contents of the drug container. For example, the ampule containing Dolophine (Figure 11.6) actually contains approximately 1.2 mL. You must inject only _____ mL of Dolophine to accurately execute the physician's order. The excess 0.2 mL of solution should be discarded.

one

---- **14** ----

You will need to calculate a parenteral drug dosage when the prescribed dosage is different from the _____ dosage. Use the ratio-and-proportion method to calculate the amount to administer.

available

---- **15** ----

Let's review the three steps of the ratio-and-proportion method of calculation. First, select two equal ratios and write them as a proportion, labeled "known" ratio and "want-to-know" ratio.

dosage strength
prescribed dosage

The ______ ______ becomes the "known" ratio and the ______ ______ becomes the "want-to-know" ratio. Second, write the units in proportional form and then write the quantities in proportional form. Third, multiply the means and extremes and solve for the unknown quantity.

16

150 mg/mL

Look at the medication label in Figure 11.7. The dosage strength for Cleocin is ______.

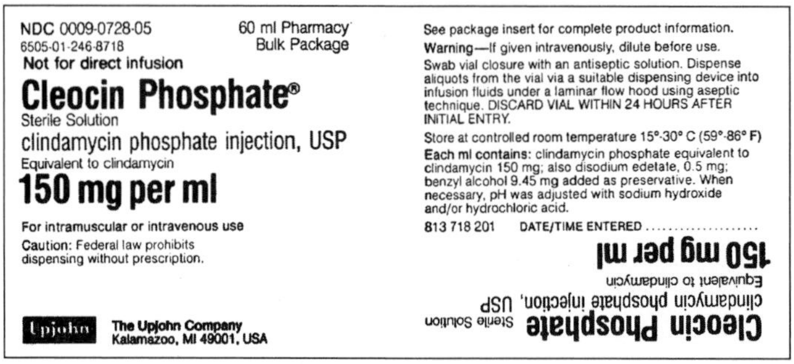

NDC 0009-0728-05
6505-01-246-8718
60 ml Pharmacy Bulk Package
Not for direct infusion
Cleocin Phosphate®
Sterile Solution
clindamycin phosphate injection, USP
Equivalent to clindamycin
150 mg per ml
For intramuscular or intravenous use
Caution: Federal law prohibits dispensing without prescription.
Upjohn
The Upjohn Company
Kalamazoo, MI 49001, USA
See package insert for complete product information.
Warning—If given intravenously, dilute before use.
Swab vial closure with an antiseptic solution. Dispense aliquots from the vial via a suitable dispensing device into infusion fluids under a laminar flow hood using aseptic technique. DISCARD VIAL WITHIN 24 HOURS AFTER INITIAL ENTRY.
Store at controlled room temperature 15°-30° C (59°-86° F)
Each ml contains: clindamycin phosphate equivalent to clindamycin 150 mg; also disodium edetate, 0.5 mg; benzyl alcohol 9.45 mg added as preservative. When necessary, pH was adjusted with sodium hydroxide and/or hydrochloric acid.
813 718 201
DATE/TIME ENTERED ....
150 mg per ml
Equivalent to clindamycin
clindamycin phosphate injection, USP
Cleocin Phosphate
Sterile Solution

FIGURE 11.7

17

Using Figure 11.7, let's determine the amount of medication you will administer for the order, "Cleocin 225 mg IM now."

known ratio = want-to-know ratio

mg:mL = mg:mL ⟵ **units in proportional form**

$150:1 = 225:x$ ⟵ **quantities in proportional form**

$150:1 = 225:x$ ⟵ **multiply means and extremes**

$150x = 225$

$\frac{\cancel{150}x}{\cancel{150}} = \frac{225}{150}$ ⟵ **cancel**

$x = 1.5\text{ mL}$

1.5 mL

You will administer ______ of Cleocin.

REMEMBER

The average volume of drug administered SQ is 1 mL or less, while the average volume injected IM is usually 1–3 mL for a single dose.

IF THE AMOUNT OF DRUG YOU CALCULATED TO BE GIVEN EXCEEDS THIS AMOUNT, RECHECK YOUR CALCULATIONS.

18

Now You Try It

Determine the volume of medication you will administer using the labels provided.

a. Look at Figure 11.8. The order reads: Depo-Medrol 60 mg IM now. You will administer _____.

New Formula
Depo-Medrol®
Sterile Aqueous Suspension
sterile methylprednisolone
acetate suspension, USP
80 mg per mL

5 mL
For IM, intrasynovial and soft tissue injection only.
NOT for I.V. use.
Contains Benzyl Alcohol as a Preservative.
See package insert for complete product information
Shake well immediately before using.
811 883 203
The Upjohn Company
Kalamazoo, MI 49001, USA

FIGURE 11.8

a. mg:mL = mg:mL

$$80:1 = 60:x$$

$$\frac{80x}{80} = \frac{60}{80}$$

$$x = 0.75 \text{ mL}$$

b. Look at Figure 11.9. The order reads: atropine 0.3 mg IM @ 0800. You will administer _____.

Store at 59° to 86°F (15° to 30°C)
Usual Adult Dose—0.75 to 1.5 mL injected subcutaneously, intramuscularly, or slowly intravenously. See literature.
Each mL contains Atropine Sulfate, 0.4 mg with Chlorobutanol (Chloroform Derivative) 0.5 percent.
WV 6730 AMX
Eli Lilly & Co., Indianapolis, IN 46285, U.S.A.

APPROXIMATE EQUIVALENTS
0.4 mL = 0.16 mg
0.5 mL = 0.2 mg
0.6 mL = 0.24 mg
0.8 mL = 0.32 mg
1.25 mL = 0.4 mg
1.6 mL = 0.5 mg
2.5 mL = 0.65 mg
3.1 mL = 1.0 mg
mL = 1.25 mg

Exp. Date/Control No.

NDC 0002-1675-01
20 mL   VIAL No. 419
℞
POISON   *Lilly*

ATROPINE
SULFATE
INJECTION, USP
0.4 mg per mL
CAUTION—Federal (U.S.A.) law prohibits dispensing without prescription.

FIGURE 11.9

b. mg:mL = mg:mL

$$0.4:1 = 0.3:x$$

$$\frac{0.4x}{0.4} = \frac{0.3}{0.4}$$

$$x = 0.75 \text{ mL}$$

c. U:ml = U:ml

10,000:1 = 7200:x

$$\frac{10000x}{10000} = \frac{7200}{10000}$$

x = 0.72 mL

d. mg:mL = mg:mL

300:2 = 200:x

$$\frac{300x}{300} = \frac{400}{300}$$

x = 1.33 mL

e. U:mL = U:mL

300000:1 = 250000:x

$$\frac{300000x}{300000} = \frac{250000}{300000}$$

x = 0.83 mL

same

c. Look at Figure 11.10. The order reads: heparin 7200 U **SQ** b.i.d. You will administer _____.

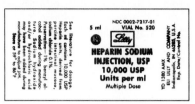

FIGURE 11.10

d. Look at Figure 11.11. The order reads: Tagamet 200 mg IM q.6h. You will administer _____.

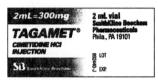

FIGURE 11.11

e. Look at Figure 11.12. The order reads: Crysticillin 250,000 U IM now. You will administer _____.

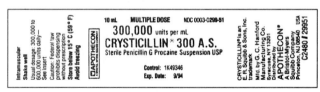

FIGURE 11.12

REMEMBER

Check all your answers by substituting the unknown quantity *x* with your answer. The product of the means should equal the product of the extremes.

── **19** ──

Occasionally the prescribed dosage and the available dosage are in different units or systems of measurement. To calculate the volume of measurement to administer, the prescribed dosage and the available dosage must be in the _____ units of measurement.

20

Look at the label in Figure 11.13. Let's determine the number of milliliters you will administer for the order, "Kantrex 0.4 g IM now." First, convert 0.4 g to an equivalent amount of milligrams, using the ratio-and-proportion method. Refer to the Equivalency Tables on the inside front and back covers.

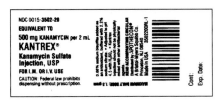

FIGURE 11.13

known ratio = want-to-know ratio

$g:mg = g:mg$ ⟵ units in proportional form

$1:1000 = 0.4:x$ ⟵ quantities in proportional form

$1:1000 = 0.4:x$ ⟵ multiply means and extremes

$x = 400$ mg

Therefore 0.4 g is equivalent to 400 mg.

21

Once the prescribed amount and the available amount are in the same units of measurement, you can easily determine the volume in milliliters you will administer. Remember to substitute _____ for 0.4 g in the medication order.

400 mg

known ratio = want-to-know ratio

$mg:mL = mg:mL$ ⟵ units in proportional form

$500:2 = 400:x$ ⟵ quantities in proportional form

$500:2 = 400:x$ ⟵ multiply means and extremes

$500x = 800$

$$\frac{\cancel{500}x}{\cancel{500}} = \frac{\cancel{800}}{\cancel{500}} \quad \longleftarrow \text{ cancel}$$

$$x = 1.6 \text{ mL}$$

You will administer _____ of Kantrex.

1.6 mL

a. g:mg = g:mg

1:1000 = 0.5:x

x = 500 mg

mg:mL = mg:mL

500:2 = 600:x

$$\frac{\cancel{500}x}{\cancel{500}} = \frac{\cancel{1200}}{\cancel{500}}$$

x = 2.4 mL

2.4 mL streptomycin

22

Now You Try It

Determine the volume of medication you will administer using the given available dosages. Round your answers to the nearest tenth.

a. The available dose is streptomycin 0.5 g/2 mL. The order reads: streptomycin 600 mg IM now. You will administer _____.

b. mg:mcg = mg:mcg

1:1000 = 0.2:x

x = 200 mcg

mcg:mL = mcg:mL

200:1 = 150:x

$$\frac{\cancel{200}x}{\cancel{200}} = \frac{150}{200}$$

x = 0.8 mL

0.8 mL Robinul

b. The available dose is Robinul 0.2 mg/mL. The order reads: Robinul 150 mcg IM now. You will administer _____.

c. gr:mg = gr:mg

$$1:60 = \frac{1}{6}:x$$

$$x = \frac{\cancel{60}^{10}}{1} \times \frac{1}{\cancel{6}}$$

x = 10 mg

mg:cc = mg:cc

15:1 = 10:x

$$\frac{\cancel{15}x}{\cancel{15}} = \frac{10}{15}$$

x = 0.7 cc

0.7 cc morphine

c. The available dose is morphine 15 mg/cc. The order reads: morphine gr $\frac{1}{6}$ IM q.3–4h p.r.n. pain. You will administer _____.

d. The available dose is codeine gr $\frac{1}{4}$ per cc. The order reads: codeine 30 mg IM q.4–6h p.r.n. pain. You will administer _____ .

Reconstituting Powdered Parenteral Drugs

--------- **23** ---------

Some parenteral medications are prepared in powdered form to help maintain the potency and shelf life of the medication. These medications, as with oral powdered drugs, must be _____ , or reconstituted, before use.

--------- **24** ---------

To reconstitute a powdered medication for parenteral use, a _____ solvent must be added to the container. The solvents commonly used for this purpose include sterile water, bacteriostatic water, and sterile 0.9% sodium chloride solution. The medication label or package insert will list the directions for reconstitution and will designate the type and amount of solvent.

--------- **25** ---------

To begin the reconstitution process, find the directions on the medication _____ or the _____ _____ .

--------- **26** ---------

Examine Figure 11.14 (see page 154). Find and read the directions for reconstitution for IM use. The amount and type of solvent to add is _____ .

d. gr:mg = gr:mg

$1:60 = \frac{1}{4}:x$

$x = \frac{\overset{15}{\cancel{60}}}{1} \times \frac{1}{\cancel{4}}$

$x = 15$ mg

mg:cc = mg:cc

$15:1 = 30:x$

$\frac{\cancel{15}x}{\cancel{15}} = \frac{30}{15}$

$x = 2$ cc

2 cc codeine

liquified

sterile

label
package insert

2.5 mL Sterile Water

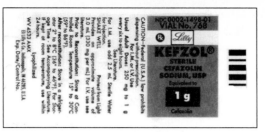

FIGURE 11.14

27
---

reconstituting

330 mg/mL

After liquifying, or _____, the medication, you will determine the dosage strength of the prepared solution. In Figure 11.14, the dosage strength for Kefzol is _____.

> **REMEMBER**
>
> **Read all the directions for reconstitution carefully.**

28
---

mg:mL = mg:mL

330:1 = 500:x

330:1 = 500:x

330x = 500

$$\frac{330x}{330} = \frac{500}{330}$$

x = 1.5 mL

1.5 mL Kefzol

Next, calculate the amount of medication to administer. Using Figure 11.14, determine the amount of medication you will administer for the order, "Kefzol 500 mg IM q.6h." Round your answer to the nearest tenth.
You will administer _____.

29
---

24 hours
room temperature

To complete the reconstitution process, circle or write the dosage strength of the prepared solution on the medication label. Write on the label the date and time the drug will expire after reconstitution. The directions regarding the length of potency of Kefzol after reconstitution state that it must be used within _____ _____, if kept at _____ _____.

REMEMBER

When reconstituting a powdered medication:
* ★ Read the directions.
* ★ Determine the amount and type of solvent.
* ★ Determine the dosage strength of the liquified medication.
* ★ Calculate the volume of medication you will administer.
* ★ Indicate the medication's expiration date by writing the date and time of reconstitution with your initials on the medication label.

30

Now You Try It

Record the following information about reconstitution for each label provided. Determine the amount of medicine you will administer for each medication. Round your answers to the nearest tenth.

NDC 0009-0698-01
8–125 mg doses

Solu-Medrol®1 gram*
Sterile Powder

methylprednisolone sodium
succinate for injection, USP

For intramuscular or
intravenous use

Caution: Federal law prohibits
dispensing without prescription.

Upjohn

See package insert for complete product information.
Store at controlled room temperature 15°-30° C (59°-86° F)
Reconstitute with 16.0 ml Bacteriostatic Water for injection with Benzyl Alcohol. **When reconstituted as directed each 16.0 ml** contains: *Methylprednisolone sodium succinate equivalent to 1 gram methylprednisolone (62.5 mg per ml).
Store solution at controlled room temperature 15°-30° F (59°-86° F) and use within 48 hours after mixing.
Lyophilized in container   812 374 201
Reconstituted: ....

The Upjohn Company
Kalamazoo, MI 49001, USA

FIGURE 11.15

a. Look at Figure 11.15. Determine the

type of solvent _____

amount of solvent _____

dosage strength _____

length of potency _____

The order reads: Solu-Medrol 80 mg IM. You will administer _____.

a. Bacteriostatic Water
16 mL
62.5 mg/mL
48 hours
mg:mL = mg:mL

$62.5{:}1 = 80{:}x$

$\dfrac{62.5x}{62.5} = \dfrac{80}{62.5}$

$x = 1.3$ mL

1.3 mL Solu-Medrol

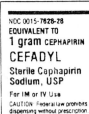

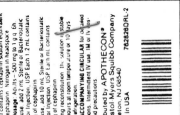

...olu-Medrol provides a space ...the drug was reconstituted. ...nitials.

not listed on label,
need to read
package insert

g:mg = g:mg

1:1000 = 0.5:x

x = 500 mg

mg:mL = mg:mL

250:1 = 500:x

$\frac{250x}{250} = \frac{500}{250}$

x = 2 mL

2 mL Nafcillin

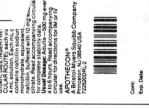

NAFCILLIN SODIUM FOR INJECTION, USP

FIGURE 11.16

b. Examine Figure 11.16. Determine the

type of solvent _____

amount of solvent _____

dosage strength _____

length of potency _____

The order reads: Nafcillin 0.5 g IM b.i.d. You will administer _____.

c. sterile or
Bacteriostatic Water

2 mL

500 mg/1.2 mL

12 hours at room
temperature
10 days refrigerated

mg:mL = mg:mL

500:1.2 = 625:x

$\frac{500x}{500} = \frac{750}{500}$

x = 1.5 mL

1.5 mL Cefadyl

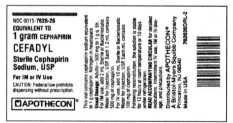

FIGURE 11.17

c. Examine Figure 11.17. Determine the

type of solvent _____

amount of solvent _____

dosage strength _____

length of potency _____

The order reads: Cefadyl 750 mg IM now. You will administer _____.

☆ What You've Achieved!

★ You can calculate dosages for parenteral medication.

★ You always remember to convert all dosages to the same system of measurement and all units to the same size.

★ You know how to reconstitute and label parenteral medications supplied in a powdered form.

Terrific! What you've learned in this chapter will help you calculate, prepare, and administer parenteral medications. Before moving forward, take the review test to demonstrate your mastery of dosage calculations for parentral medications. If you get more than two wrong in section A or one wrong in section B, consider reading that portion of the chapter again.

Review Test

Professional literature stipulates the following medications may be given IM. However, the trend today, especially in the hospital setting, is to use the IV route. The following problems use the IM route for practice purposes even though the medications may be more frequently administered IV.

—————————————————— **A** ——————————————————

Determine the amount of medication you will administer using the given available dosage or medication label provided. Round your answer to the nearest tenth.

1. Examine Figure 11.18. The order reads: Compazine 6 mg IM now. You will administer _____.

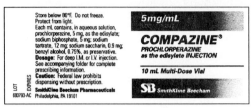

FIGURE 11.18

2. Examine Figure 11.19. The order reads: Vistaril 75 mg IM q.6h p.r.n. nausea. You will administer _____.

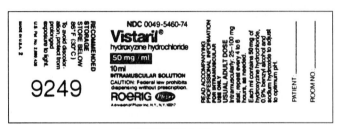

FIGURE 11.19

3. The available dosage is Demerol 100 mg/mL. The order reads: Demerol 75 mg IM q.4h p.r.n. You will administer _____.

4. The available dosage is Levo-Dromoran 2 mg/mL. The order reads: Levo-Dromoran 1.5 mg IM. You will administer _____.

5. The available dosage is vitamin B_{12} 120 mcg/mL. The order reads: vitamin B_{12} 0.16 mg IM now. You will administer _____.

6. The available dosage is Zantac 25 mg/mL. The order reads: Zantac 0.05 g IM. You will administer _____.

7. The available dosage is Seconal gr $\frac{3}{4}$/mL. The order reads: Seconal 100 mg IM h.s. p.r.n. You will administer _____.

8. The available dosage is digoxin 250 mcg/cc. The order reads: digoxin 0.125 mg now. You will administer _____.

9. The available dosage is penicillin G 6,000,000 U/10 mL. The order reads: penicillin G 1,200,000 U IM. You will administer _____.

10. The available dosage is calcitonin 200 U/mL. The order reads: calcitonin 150 U SQ. You will administer _____.

11. The available dosage is morphine 10 mg/cc. The order reads: morphine gr $\frac{1}{10}$ IM q.3h p.r.n. You will administer _____.

─────────────────────────── **B** ───────────────────────────

Record the following reconstitution information. Use the labels to determine the amount of medication you will administer. Round your answers to the nearest tenth.

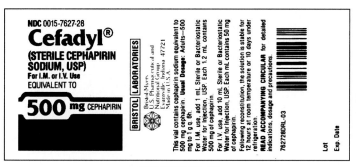

FIGURE 11.20

12. Examine Figure 11.20. Determine the

types of solvent _____

amount of solvent _____

dosage strength _____

length of potency _____

The order reads: Cefadyl 0.25 g IM. You will administer _____.

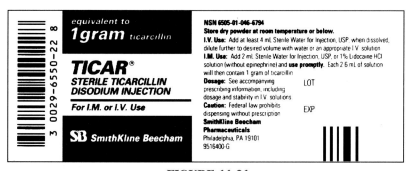

FIGURE 11.21

13. Examine Figure 11.21. Determine the

type of solvent _____

amount of solvent _____

dosage strength _____

length of potency _____

The order reads: Ticar 0.5 g IM now. You will administer _____.

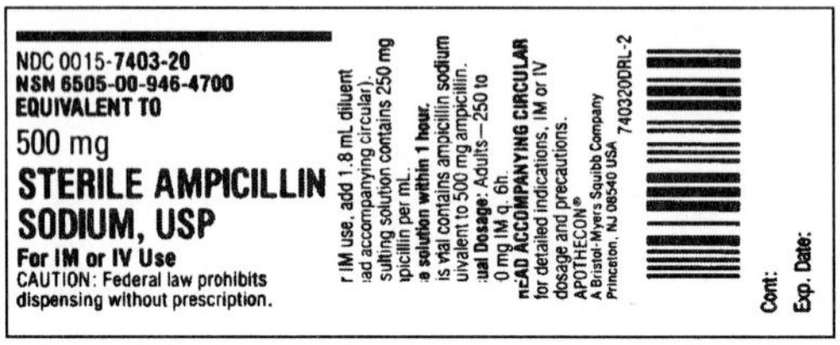

NDC 0015-**7403-20**
NSN 6505-00-946-4700
EQUIVALENT TO
500 mg
STERILE AMPICILLIN SODIUM, USP
For IM or IV Use
CAUTION: Federal law prohibits dispensing without prescription.

r IM use, add 1.8 mL diluent (ied accompanying circular). sulting solution contains 250 mg ipicillin per mL. **a solution within 1 hour.** is vial contains ampicillin sodium uivalent to 500 mg ampicillin. ual Dosage: Adults—250 to 0 mg IM q. 6h. mcAD ACCOMPANYING CIRCULAR for detailed indications, IM or IV dosage and precautions. APOTHECON® A Bristol-Myers Squibb Company Princeton, NJ 08540 USA 740320DRL-2

Cont:
Exp. Date:

FIGURE 11.22

14. Examine Figure 11.22. Determine the

type of solvent _____

amount of solvent _____

dosage strength _____

length of potency _____

The order reads ampicillin 450 mg IM q.6h. You will administer _____.

NDC 0015-**7226-28**
EQUIVALENT TO
2 gram NAFCILLIN
NAFCILLIN SODIUM
FOR INJECTION, USP
Buffered–For IM or IV Use
CAUTION: Federal law prohibits dispensing without prescription.
APOTHECON
A BRISTOL-MYERS SQUIBB COMPANY ®

When reconstituted with 6.6 mL diluent, (SEE INSERT-INTRAMUS-CULAR ROUTE), each vial contains 8 mL solution. Each mL of solution contains nafcillin sodium, as the monohydrate, equivalent to 250 mg nafcillin, buffered with 10 mg sodium citrate. Read accompanying circular for complete stability data. Usual Dosage: Adults—500 mg every 4 to 6 hours. Read accompanying circular for directions for IM or IV use. APOTHECON® A Bristol-Myers Squibb Company Princeton, NJ 08540 USA 726620DRL-2

Cont:
Exp. Date:

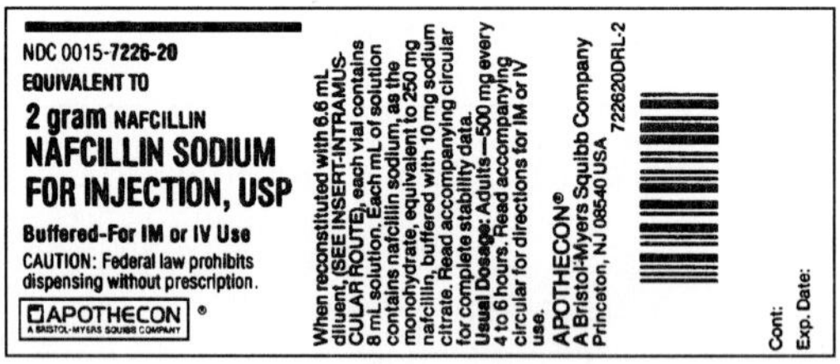

FIGURE 11.23

15. Examine Figure 11.23. Determine the

type of solvent _____

amount of solvent _____

dosage strength _____

The order reads: nafcillin 375 mg IM q.6h. You will administer _____.

Answers for Review Test

1. mg:mL = mg:mL

$$5{:}1 = 6{:}x$$

$$\frac{\cancel{5}x}{\cancel{5}} = \frac{6}{5}$$

$$x = 1.2 \text{ mL}$$

1.2 mL Compazine

2. mg:mL = mg:mL

$$50{:}1 = 75{:}x$$

$$\frac{\cancel{50}x}{\cancel{50}} = \frac{75}{50}$$

$$x = 1.5 \text{ mL}$$

1.5 mL Vistaril

3. mg:mL = mg:mL

$$100{:}1 = 75{:}x$$

$$\frac{\cancel{100}x}{\cancel{100}} = \frac{75}{100}$$

$$x = 0.8 \text{ mL}$$

0.8 mL Demerol

4. mg:mL = mg:mL

$$2{:}1 = 1.5{:}x$$

$$\frac{\cancel{2}x}{\cancel{2}} = \frac{1.5}{2}$$

$$x = 0.8 \text{ mL}$$

0.8 mL Levo-Dromoran

5. mg:mcg = mg:mcg

$$1{:}1000 = 0.16{:}x$$

$$x = 160 \text{ mcg}$$

mcg:mL = mcg:mL

$$120{:}1 = 160{:}x$$

$$\frac{\cancel{120}x}{\cancel{120}} = \frac{\cancel{160}}{\cancel{120}}$$

$$x = 1.3 \text{ mL}$$

1.3 mL vitamin B_{12}

6. g:mg = g:mg

$$1{:}1000 = 0.05{:}x$$

$$x = 50 \text{ mg}$$

mg:mL = mg:mL

$$25{:}1 = 50{:}x$$

$$\frac{\cancel{25}x}{\cancel{25}} = \frac{50}{25}$$

$$x = 2 \text{ mL}$$

2 mL Zantac

7. gr:mg = gr:mg

$$1{:}60 = \frac{3}{4}{:}x$$

$$x = 45 \text{ mcg}$$

mg:mL = mg:mL

$$45{:}1 = 100{:}x$$

$$\frac{\cancel{45}x}{\cancel{45}} = \frac{100}{45}$$

$$x = 2.2 \text{ mL}$$

2.2 mL Seconal

8. mcg:mg = mcg:mg

$$1000{:}1 = x{:}0.125$$

$$x = 125 \text{ mcg}$$

mcg:cc = mcg:cc

$$250{:}1 = 125{:}x$$

$$\frac{\cancel{250}x}{\cancel{250}} = \frac{125}{250}$$

$$x = 0.5 \text{ cc}$$

0.5 cc digoxin

9. U:mL = U:mL

$$6{,}000{,}000{:}10 = 1{,}200{,}000{:}x$$

$$\frac{\cancel{6000000}x}{\cancel{6000000}} = \frac{\cancel{12000000}}{\cancel{6000000}}$$

$$x = 2 \text{ mL}$$

2 mL penicillin G

10. U:mL = U:mL

200:1 = 150:x

$\dfrac{200x}{200} = \dfrac{150}{200}$

$x = 0.75$ mL

0.8 mL calcitonin

11. gr:mg = gr:mg

1:60 = $\dfrac{1}{10}$:x

$x = 6$ mg

mg:cc = mg:cc

10:1 = 6:x

$\dfrac{10x}{10} = \dfrac{6}{10}$

$x = 0.6$ cc

0.6 cc morphine

12. Sterile or Bacteriostatic water

1 mL

500 mg/1.2 mL

12 hours at room temperature, 10 days under refrigeration

g:mg = g:mg

1:1000 = 0.25:x

$x = 250$ mg

mg:mL = mg:mL

500:1.2 = 250:x

$\dfrac{500x}{500} = \dfrac{300}{500}$

$x = 0.6$ mL

0.6 mL Cefadyl

---

13. Sterile water

2 mL

1 g/2.6 mL

Use promptly

g:mL = g:mL

1:2.6 = 0.5:x

$x = 1.3$ mL

1.3 mL Ticar

14. unknown diluent

1.8 mL

250 mg/1 mL

use solution within 1 hour

mg:mL = mg:mL

250:1 = 450:x

$\dfrac{250x}{250} = \dfrac{450}{250}$

$x = 1.8$ mL

1.8 mL ampicillin

15. unknown diluent

6.6 mL

250 mg/mL

mg:mL = mg:mL

250:1 = 375:x

$\dfrac{250x}{250} = \dfrac{375}{250}$

$x = 1.5$ mL

1.5 mL nafcillin

Syringes

Objectives

When you finish this chapter, you will be able to:

★ State the uses of standard 3-cc, tuberculin, and insulin syringes.

★ Read the calibrations and measure correct dosages using standard 3-cc, tuberculin, or insulin syringes.

★ Understand the method used to mix two parenteral medications in one syringe.

★ Read the calibrations and measure correct dosages for two medications combined in one syringe.

Chapter Outline

★ The Standard 3-cc Syringe
★ The Prefilled Cartridge
★ The Tuberculin Syringe
★ The Insulin Syringe
★ Mixing Two Medications
★ Combining Two Kinds of Insulin

Introduction

You will need to use a variety of syringes when administering medications parenterally. The standard 3-cc, tuberculin, and insulin syringes are the most frequently used. A small number of medications are packaged in **prefilled** single-use **cartridges**. The type of syringe you select is determined by the **amount** of medication to be given and the administration **route** (IM, SQ, or IV).

The volume of standard 3-cc and tuberculin syringes is calibrated in cubic centimeters (cc) and minims (♏). The volume of prefilled cartridges is calibrated in cubic centimeters only. Insulin syringe volumes are calibrated in units. Each unit is equal to a hundredth of a cc.

The standard 3-cc syringe has a comparatively large capacity and is calibrated in tenths (0.1) of a cc. The prefilled cartridge is also calibrated in tenths of a cc but has a smaller capacity of 1 to 2.5 cc. The tuberculin syringe has a capacity of only 1 cc. It is calibrated in tenths (0.1) and hundredths (0.01) of a cc. Insulin syringes are calibrated in units. The U-100 insulin syringe has a capacity of 100 units, while the Lo-Dose® insulin syringe has a 50-unit capacity. The calibrations for all syringes start at zero and go to the capacity of the specific syringe.

The Standard 3-cc Syringe

────────────────── **1** ──────────────────

tuberculin
insulin

The three common types of syringes are standard 3-cc, _____, and _____.

────────────────── **2** ──────────────────

IM

The **standard 3-cc** syringe is a multiple-use syringe. You will use this type of syringe to administer most intramuscular (_____) injections.

────────────────── **3** ──────────────────

tenths

The calibrations on a standard 3-cc syringe are subdivided into _____ of a cc. Accordingly, you need to round off dosage calculations to the nearest tenth when using a standard 3-cc syringe.

────────────────── **4** ──────────────────

known
want-to-know

mg:cc = mg:cc
$25:1 = 35:x$

$\dfrac{25x}{25} = \dfrac{35}{25}$

$x = 1.4$ cc
1.4 cc Phenergan

You may have to convert between systems of measurement to determine the amount of medication to administer parenterally. To review, first select two equal ratios and write them as a proportion, labeled "_____" ratio and "_____ ____ _____" ratio. Next write the units in proportional form; then write the quantities in proportional form. Finally, multiply the means and extremes and solve for the unknown quantity.

────────────────── **5** ──────────────────

Let's consider the medication order, Phenergan 35 mg IM q.4h p.r.n. nausea. If Phenergan 25 mg/cc is available, the amount you will administer is _____.

6

Figure 12.1 shows the amount you will draw into a standard 3-cc syringe to administer the required dosage. The amount of Phenergan in the syringe is ———————.

1.4 cc Phenergan

1.4cc

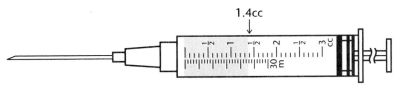

FIGURE 12.1

DID YOU NOTICE?

The larger calibration marks identify the zero, one-half, and full cc measures. The smaller calibration marks identify tenths of a cc.

7

Now You Try It

Solve the following dosage problems. Place an arrow against each sample standard 3-cc syringe to indicate the amount of medication you will draw into the syringe. Round to the nearest tenth.

REMEMBER

The first calibration mark on all syringes is zero.

a. The available dosage is Compazine 10 mg/2 mL. The drug order reads: Compazine 8 mg IM q.4–6h p.r.n. nausea. You will administer ———————.

a. mg:mL = mg:mL

$$10{:}2 = 8{:}x$$

$$\frac{10x}{10} = \frac{16}{10}$$

$$x = 1.6 \text{ mL}$$

1.6 mL Compazine

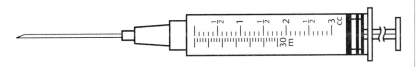

FIGURE 12.2

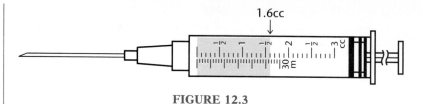

1.6cc

FIGURE 12.3

b. mg:mL = mg:mL

300:2 = 225:x

$$\frac{300x}{300} = \frac{450}{300}$$

x = 1.5 mL
1.5 mL Tagamet

b. The available dosage is Tagamet 300 mg/2 mL. The drug order reads: Tagamet 225 mg IM b.i.d. You will administer _____.

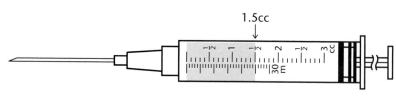

FIGURE 12.4

1.5cc

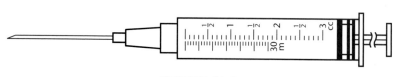

FIGURE 12.5

c. g:mg = g:mg

1:1000 = 0.125:x

x = 125 mg

mg:mL = mg:mL

125:1 = 150:x

$$\frac{125x}{125} = \frac{150}{125}$$

x = 1.2 mL
1.2 mL Terramycin

c. The available dosage is Terramycin 0.125 g/mL. The order reads: Terramycin 150 mg IM q.12h. You will administer _____.

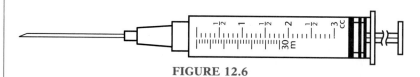

FIGURE 12.6

1.2cc

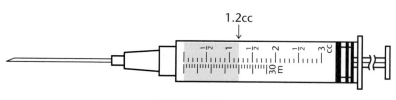

FIGURE 12.7

d. The available dosage is gentamicin 80 mg/2 mL. The drug order reads: gentamicin 70 mg IM q.6h. You will administer _____.

d. mg:mL = mg:mL

$$80:2 = 70:x$$

$$\frac{\cancel{80}x}{\cancel{80}} = \frac{\cancel{140}}{\cancel{80}}$$

$$x = 1.75 \text{ mL}$$
or 1.8 mL

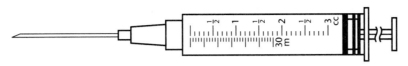

FIGURE 12.8

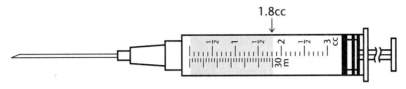

FIGURE 12.9

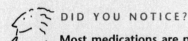
DID YOU NOTICE?

Most medications are prepared and labeled in mL measures, while most syringes are calibrated in cc's.

The Prefilled Cartridge

8

Some parenteral medications are available in prefilled single dose cartridges. The cartridges are usually _____ in capacity, with the drug and dosage clearly marked.

1–2.5 cc

9

Like an ampule (see Chapter 11), a prefilled cartridge usually contains 0.1–0.2 cc of excess medication. The excess medication must be _____ before the drug is administered. You discard the unneeded portion of the medication by ejecting the excess out of the cartridge before injecting the patient.

discarded

10

0.2 cc

For example, in the order, morphine 10 mg IM q.3h p.r.n., the cartridge available reads: morphine 10 mg/cc. The amount of prepared solution in the cartridge is 1.2 cc. For an accurate dosage of morphine to be given, _____, must be discarded.

REMEMBER

Administer the exact volume of medication needed to execute the physician's order.

11

mg:mL = mg:mL

50:1 = 35:x

$\dfrac{50x}{50} = \dfrac{35}{50}$

x = 0.7 mL
0.7 mL Demerol

Drugs commonly packaged in a prefilled cartridge include morphine, Demerol, Mepergan, codeine, Toradol, and aqueous penicillin. In the order, Demerol 35 mg IM for pain, the cartridge available reads: Demerol 50 mg/mL. You will administer _____.

12

Now You Try It

Calculate the amount of medication you will administer using the available dosage. Round to the nearest tenth.

a. mg:mL = mg:mL

60:2 = 45:x

$\dfrac{60x}{60} = \dfrac{90x}{60}$

x = 1.5 mL
1.5 mL Toradol

a. The available dosage is Toradol cartridge, 60 mg/2 mL. The order reads: Toradol 45 mg IM q.6h. You will administer _____.

b. mg:mL = mg:mL

100:1 = 65:x

$\dfrac{100x}{100} = \dfrac{65}{100}$

x = 0.65 mL

or 0.7 mL
0.7 mL meperidine

b. The available dosage is meperidine cartridge, 100 mg/mL. The order reads: meperidine 65 mg IM q.4h p.r.n. pain. You will administer _____.

The Tuberculin Syringe

13

0.1
0.01

The tuberculin syringe is a 1 cc syringe calibrated in _____ and _____ cc subdivisions.

14

When using a tuberculin syringe, calculate dosages to the thousandth and round off to the nearest _____.

hundredth (0.01)

15

You will use tuberculin syringes to administer drug dosages of _____ or less. Drugs administered by a tuberculin syringe include heparin, tetanus toxoid, and allergen extracts for skin tests. Tuberculin syringes may also be used to administer pediatric dosages.

1 cc

16

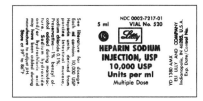

FIGURE 12.10

Consider the drug order, heparin 7000 U SQ. Consult the medication label shown in Figure 12.10 and calculate the dosage. You will administer _____. Place an arrow on the sample tuberculin syringe to indicate the amount of medication you will draw into the syringe.

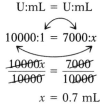

$$\text{U:mL} = \text{U:mL}$$
$$10000{:}1 = 7000{:}x$$
$$\frac{10000x}{10000} = \frac{7000}{10000}$$
$$x = 0.7 \text{ mL}$$

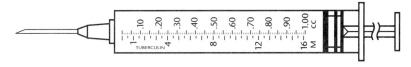

FIGURE 12.11

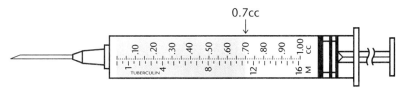

FIGURE 12.12

17

Now You Try It

Place an arrow on each sample tuberculin syringe to indicate the amount of medication you will draw into the syringe.

a. The order reads: PPD 0.2 mL ID today.

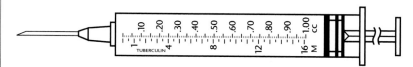

FIGURE 12.13

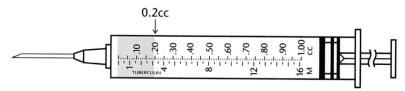

FIGURE 12.14

b. The order reads: tetanus toxoid 0.5 cc.

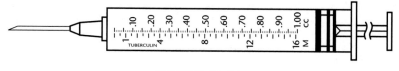

FIGURE 12.15

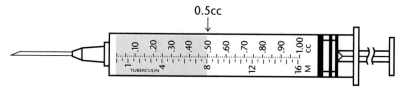

FIGURE 12.16

c. The available dosage is morphine 10 mg/mL. The order reads: morphine 6 mg **SQ** now. You will administer _____.

c. mg:mL = mg:mL

$$10:1 = 6:x$$

$$\frac{\cancel{10}x}{\cancel{10}} = \frac{6}{10}$$

$$x = 0.6 \text{ mL}$$

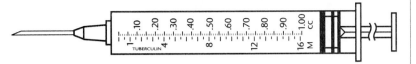

FIGURE 12.17

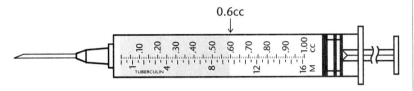

FIGURE 12.18

d. Examine Figure 12.19. The order reads: heparin 4500 U **SQ** q.12h. You will administer _____.

d. U:mL = U:mL

$$10000:1 = 4500:x$$

$$\frac{\cancel{10000}x}{\cancel{10000}} = \frac{4500}{10000}$$

$$x = 0.45 \text{ mL}$$

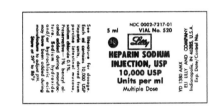

FIGURE 12.19

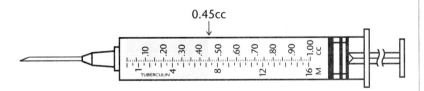

FIGURE 12.20

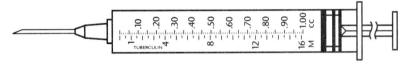

FIGURE 12.21

The Insulin Syringe

U

——————————— **18** ———————————

Insulin, which is used to treat diabetes, is measured in units, abbreviated _____. The most commonly used form of insulin is produced in concentrations (strengths) of 100 units per milliliter (U-100 insulin).

units

——————————— **19** ———————————

Insulin syringes are calibrated in _____. U-100 insulin syringes are used for the measurement and administration of **U-100** insulin. Use only insulin syringes except in emergency situations when insulin syringes are unavailable.

100 units

——————————— **20** ———————————

Examine Figure 12.22. The capacity of the standard U-100 syringe is _____.

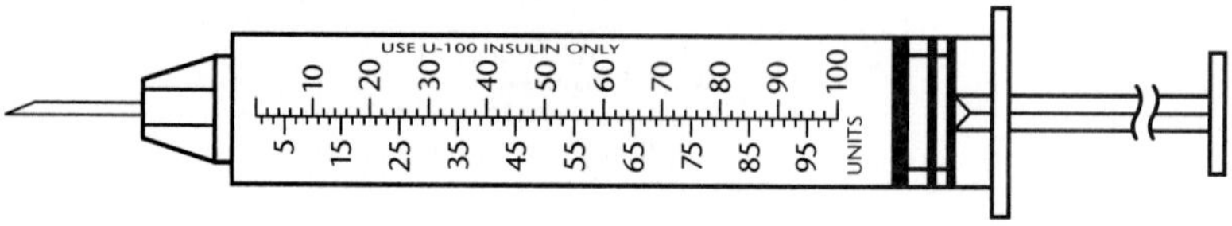

FIGURE 12.22

odd

——————————— **21** ———————————

The **standard U-100** insulin syringe is calibrated in 2-U increments, with even numbers on one side and _____ numbers on the other side of the syringe.

50-unit

——————————— **22** ———————————

The **Lo-Dose®** insulin syringe with a _____ capacity, is used for dosages less than 45 units.

5 U

——————————— **23** ———————————

Examine Figure 12.23. The syringe is calibrated in one-unit increments. Each _____ is numbered.

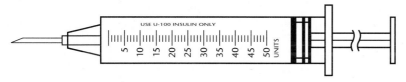

FIGURE 12.23

24

Look again at the Lo-Dose® syringe in Figure 12.23. Indicate the amount you will draw into the syringe by placing an arrow at the appropriate calibration mark for the order, NPH 35 U @ 0730.

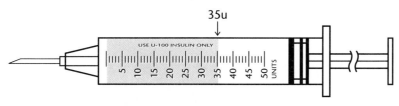

FIGURE 12.24

25

The doctor orders Humulin L 68 U SQ 0730 a.m. Consult the medication label in Figure 12.25 and indicate the measured amount on the syringe by placing an arrow at the appropriate calibration mark.

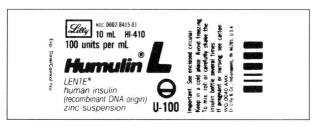

FIGURE 12.25

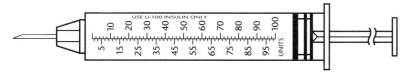

FIGURE 12.26

68u
↓

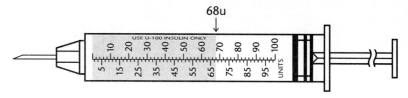

FIGURE 12.27

26

Now You Try It

Consult the medication labels. Indicate the measured amount you will draw into the syringe by placing an arrow on the appropriate mark.

REMEMBER

Use the even scale on Standard U-100 insulin syringes to measure even-numbered dosages. Use the odd scale on Standard U-100 insulin syringes to measure odd-num-bered dosages.

a.

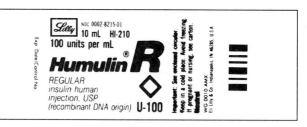

FIGURE 12.28

The order reads: Humulin R 15 U SC @ 0730.

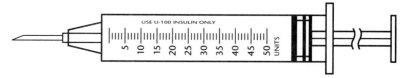

FIGURE 12.29

15u

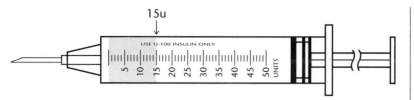

FIGURE 12.30

b.

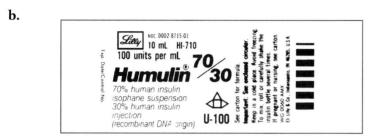

FIGURE 12.31

The order reads: Humulin 70/30 75 U SQ @ 0730.

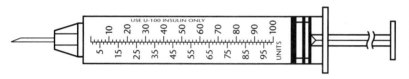

FIGURE 12.32

75u

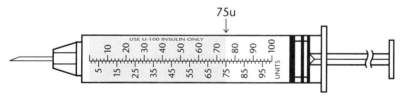

FIGURE 12.33

c.

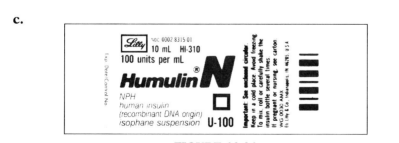

FIGURE 12.34

The order reads: Humulin N 54 U SC @ 0730.

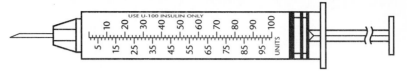

FIGURE 12.35

54u

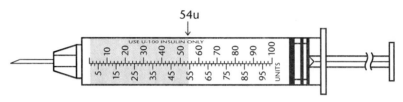

FIGURE 12.36

d.

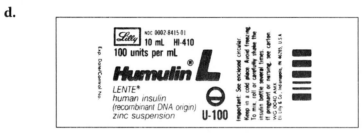

FIGURE 12.37

The order reads: Humulin L 22 U SQ @ 0730.

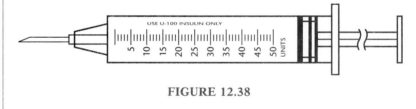

FIGURE 12.38

22u

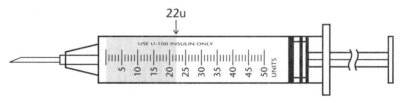

FIGURE 12.39

Mixing Two Medications

---------------------------- **27** ----------------------------

Occasionally two medications are mixed together in a syringe to avoid injecting the patient twice. It is important that the two medications be **compatible**. Compatible medications are those that do not form a **precipitate** (insoluble particles) when mixed together. You will need to consult a pharmacist or consult a drug reference to determine the _____ of two drugs.

compatibility

---------------------------- **28** ----------------------------

If a precipitate forms, indicating the medications are _____, the mixture should be discarded.

incompatible

---------------------------- **29** ----------------------------

There are several approved methods of combining two medications in one syringe. The method you will use is the easiest to learn; it involves four steps. First, draw air into the syringe equal to the volume of medication being removed from vial 1. Inject the air into vial 1. This will avoid creating a vacuum in the vial. Second, withdraw the desired amount of drug from vial 1. Remove the needle from vial _____ (see Figure 12.40a, page 178).

1

---------------------------- **30** ----------------------------

Third, insert a 25-gauge needle into the side of the rubber stopper of vial 2 to act as an air vent. Fourth, insert the needle of the syringe containing the medication from vial 1 into the center of the rubber stopper of vial 2. Invert the vial and carefully withdraw the desired volume of medication from vial 2 (see Figure 12.40b, page 178). The total volume of solution in the syringe will be the sum of _____ volumes of prescribed medication.

both

mg:mL = mg:mL

10:1 = 8:x

10x = 8

$$\frac{10x}{10} = \frac{8}{10}$$

x = 0.8 mL

0.8 mL morphine

Before you can follow the method for mixing two medications in one syringe, you will need to know the individual volumes of each prescribed dosage. Consider the medication order, morphine 8 mg IM and Phenergan 25 mg IM at 8:00 a.m. The available dosage for morphine is 10 mg/mL. Calculate the dosage of morphine. You will administer _____.

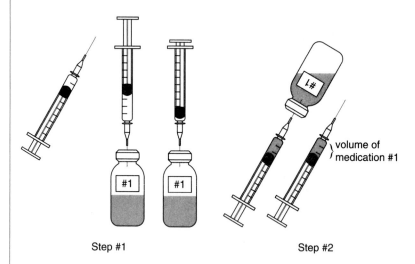

Step #1   Step #2

a. Withdrawing medication from vial #1

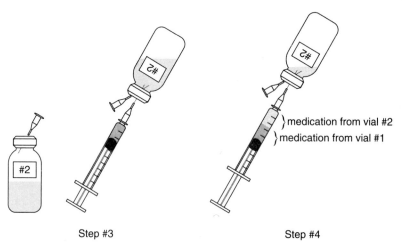

Step #3   Step #4

b. Withdrawing medication from vial #2

FIGURE 12.40

--------- **32** ---------

Now, calculate the dosage of Phenergan. The available dosage for Phenergan is 50 mg/mL. You will administer _____.

--------- **33** ---------

To mix the two medications in one syringe, withdraw the calculated volume of morphine, _____, into the syringe following the method shown in Figure 12.40a. Then, withdraw the calculated amount of Phenergan, _____, into the syringe following the method shown in Figure 12.40b. The plunger of the syringe should be moved from the 0.8 cc calibration marking to the 1.3 cc calibration marking to add 0.5 cc of Phenergan (see Figure 12.41). You will inject _____ of solution.

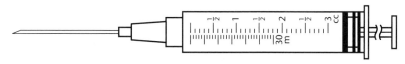

FIGURE 12.41

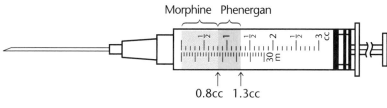

Morphine   Phenergan

0.8cc   1.3cc

FIGURE 12.42

REMEMBER

1 mL = 1 cc

--------- **34** ---------

Now You Try It

Calculate the drug dosage for each medication ordered, using the available dosage. Place arrows at the calibration marks of the sample syringe to indicate the amount of medication drawn into the syringe from both vials.

---

mg:mL = mg:mL

50:1 = 25:x

50x = 25

$\dfrac{50x}{50} = \dfrac{25}{50}$

x = 0.5 mL

0.5 mL Phenergan

0.8 mL

0.5 mL

1.3 cc

a. The drug order reads: Demerol 45 mg and Vistaril 75 mg IM now. The available dosages are Demerol 50 mg/mL and Vistaril 100 mg/2 mL. The amount of Demerol you will draw into the sample syringe is _____. The amount of Vistaril you will draw into the sample syringe is _____. The total amount of solution you will inject is _____.

a. mg:mL = mg:mL

$$50:1 = 45:x$$

$$50x = 45$$

$$\frac{50x}{50} = \frac{45}{50}$$

$$x = 0.9 \text{ mL}$$

0.9 mL Demerol

mg:mL = mg:mL

$$100:2 = 75:x$$

$$100x = 150$$

$$\frac{100x}{100} = \frac{150x}{100}$$

$$x = 1.5 \text{ mL}$$

1.5 mL Vistaril
0.9 mL + 1.5 mL =
2.4 cc

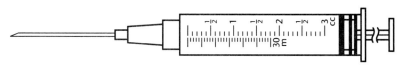

FIGURE 12.43

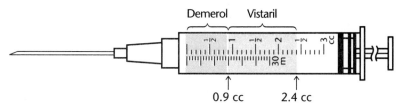

Demerol   Vistaril

0.9 cc   2.4 cc

FIGURE 12.44

b. The drug order reads: morphine 7 mg and atropine 0.5 mg IM at 10:00 a.m. The available dosages are morphine 10 mg/mL and atropine 0.4 mg/mL. The amount of morphine you will draw into the sample syringe is _____. The amount of atropine you will draw into the sample syringe is _____. The total volume of medication you will inject is _____.

b. mg:mL = mg:mL

$$10:1 = 7:x$$

$$10x = 7$$

$$\frac{10x}{10} = \frac{7}{10}$$

$$x = 0.7 \text{ mL}$$

0.7 mL morphine

mg:mL = mg:mL

$$0.4:1 = 0.5:x$$

$$0.4x = 0.5$$

$$\frac{0.4x}{0.4} = \frac{0.5}{0.4}$$

$$x = 1.25 \text{ mL or}$$
$$1.3 \text{ mL}$$

1.3 mL atropine
0.7 + 1.3 = 2 cc

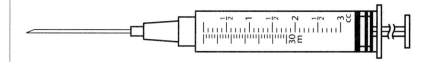

FIGURE 12.45

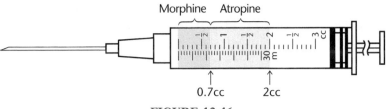

FIGURE 12.46

Combining Two Kinds of Insulin

───────────── **35** ─────────────

A fast-acting insulin (Humulin R) is often mixed with another longer-acting type of insulin (Humulin N or Humulin L) to _____ the number of injections the patient receives.

reduce

───────────── **36** ─────────────

When following the mixing procedure to combine two types of insulin in one syringe, the fast-acting insulin (Humulin R) must be withdrawn **FIRST** and, therefore, will be treated as vial _____. The longer-acting insulins will be treated as vial _____ (see Figure 12.40).

1

2

───────────── **37** ─────────────

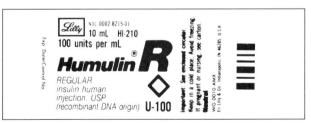

FIGURE 12.47

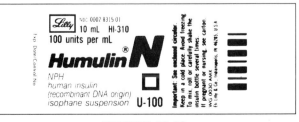

FIGURE 12.48

Consider the medication labels in Figures 12.47 and 12.48 (see page 181). The order reads: Humulin N 45 U and Humulin R 7 U SQ @ 7:30 a.m.

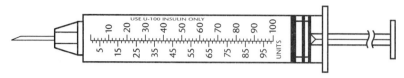

FIGURE 12.49

Place two arrows on the sample syringe to indicate the amount of Humulin R and Humulin N you will draw into the syringe.

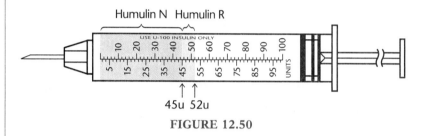

FIGURE 12.50

7 U + 45 U = 52 U

The total number of units you will inject is _____.

R E M E M B E R

Use only U-100 syringes with U-100 insulin. Match the type of syringe to the strength of insulin.

—————————————— **38** ——————————————

Humulin R

When executing the above order, _____ insulin is **ALWAYS** withdrawn into the syringe first.

—————————————— **39** ——————————————

Now You Try It

a. Consider the medication labels in Figures 12.51 and 12.52. The order reads: Humulin L 52 U & Humulin R 10 U SQ @ 0730.

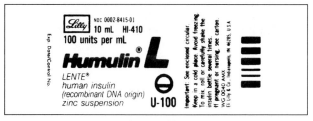

FIGURE 12.51

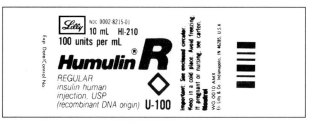

FIGURE 12.52

Place two arrows on the sample syringe to indicate the amount of Humulin R and Humulin L you will draw into the syringe.

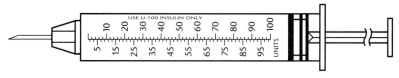

FIGURE 12.53

The total number of units you will inject is _____.

52 U + 10 U = 62 U

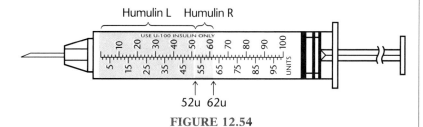

FIGURE 12.54

b. The available dosage is U-100 Regular and U-100 NPH. The order reads: Regular insulin 8 U and NPH 23 U SQ. Place two arrows on the sample syringe to indicate the amount of Regular insulin and NPH you will draw into the syringe.

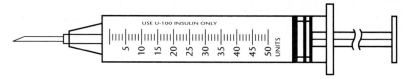

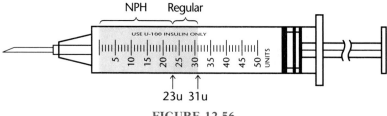

FIGURE 12.55

NPH   Regular

23u 31u

FIGURE 12.56

$8 \text{ U} + 23 \text{ U} = 31 \text{ U}$

The total number of units you will inject is _____.

⭐ What You've Achieved!

★ You know how to read and interpret the calibrations on standard 3-cc, tuberculin, standard U-100 insulin, and Lo-Dose® insulin syringes.

★ You can accurately measure one medication dosage using the standard 3-cc, tuberculin, standard U-100 insulin, and Lo-Dose® insulin syringes.

★ You have learned to measure dosages for two medications combined in one syringe.

Great work! What you've learned in this chapter will help you calculate parenteral dosages. Before moving forward, take the review test to demonstrate your mastery of reading and measuring correct dosages using syringes. If you get more than two wrong in sections A, B, and C or get section D wrong, consider rereading that portion of the chapter.

——————————————— **A** ———————————————

Complete the following statements.

1. The standard 3-cc syringe is a multiple-use syringe primarily used for _____ injections.

2. A standard 3-cc syringe has the capacity of _____ and is subdivided into _____ of a cc.

3. The tuberculin syringe is used to administer a volume less than _____.

4. A tuberculin syringe is calibrated in subdivisions of _____ and _____.

5. Tuberculin syringes are used to administer such drugs as _____, _____, and _____.

6. Insulin syringes are calibrated in _____.

7. The standard U-100 insulin syringe has a capacity of _____.

8. The _____ insulin syringe has a capacity of 50 units.

9. When mixing two insulins, the _____ insulin is drawn into the syringe first.

10. A prefilled cartridge is a _____ prepared parenteral package.

Indicate the amount you will draw into the sample syringe by placing an arrow at the appropriate mark.

11. The order reads: tetanus toxoid 0.7 cc now.

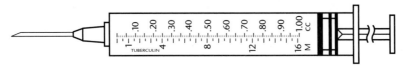

FIGURE 12.57

12. The order reads: Humulin L 38 U SQ before breakfast.

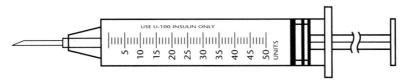

FIGURE 12.58

13. The order reads: Humulin N 71 U SQ @ 7:30 a.m.

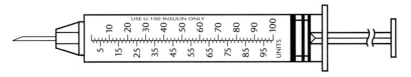

FIGURE 12.59

14. The order reads: Humulin R 5 U and Humulin L 60 U SC.

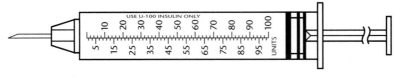

FIGURE 12.60

Calculate each dosage problem using the medication labels or available dosage. Indicate the amount you will draw into the sample syringe by placing an arrow on the appropriate calibration markings.

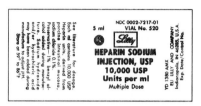

FIGURE 12.61

15. Consider Figure 12.61. The order reads: heparin 6000 U SC now. You will administer _____.

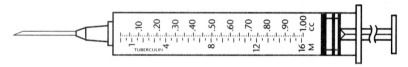

FIGURE 12.62

16. The available dosage is Compazine 10 mg/2 mL. The order reads: Compazine 4 mg IM now. You will administer _____.

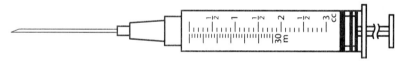

FIGURE 12.63

17. The available dosage is Depo-Provera 400 mg/mL. The order reads: Depo-Provera 500 mg IM q week. You will administer _____.

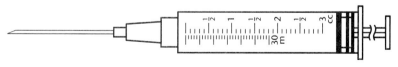

FIGURE 12.64

Calculate the drug dosage for each medication order using the available dosage. Place two arrows at the calibration markings that indicate the amount of both medications you will draw into the sample syringe.

18. The available dosages are meperidine 100 mg/mL and Robinul 0.2 mg/mL. The order reads: meperidine 85 mg and Robinul 0.1 mg IM now. The amount of meperidine you will draw into the syringe is _____.

    The amount of Robinul you will draw into the syringe is _____.

    The total amount of solution you will inject is _____.

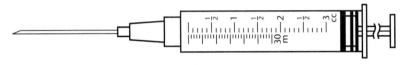

FIGURE 12.65

Answers for Review Test

1. Intramuscular   2. 3 cc, tenths (0.1)   3. 1 cc

---

4. tenths (0.1) and hundredths (0.01)   5. heparin, tetanus toxoid, allergen extract

---

6. units   7. 100 units   8. Lo-Dose®

---

9. fast-acting   10. single-dose

11.

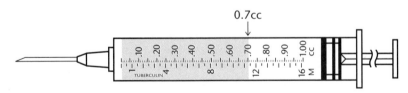

0.7cc

FIGURE 12.66

12.

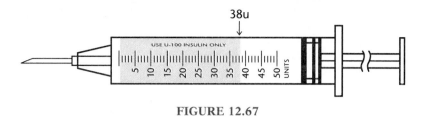

FIGURE 12.67

13.

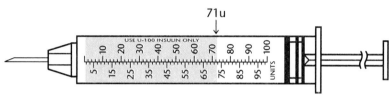

FIGURE 12.68

14.

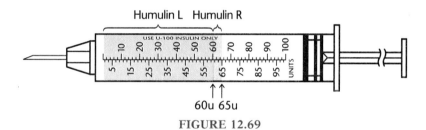

FIGURE 12.69

15. U:mL = U:mL

10000:1 = 6000:*x*

$$\frac{10000x}{10000} = \frac{6000}{10000}$$

x = 0.6 mL heparin

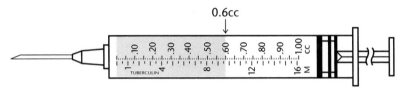

0.6cc

FIGURE 12.70

16. mg:mL = mg:mL

10:2 = 4:*x*

$$\frac{10x}{10} = \frac{8}{10}$$

x = 0.8 mL Compazine

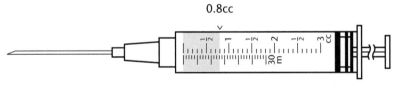

0.8cc

FIGURE 12.71

17. mg:mL = mg:mL

$$400{:}1 = 500{:}x$$

$$\frac{\cancel{400}x}{\cancel{400}} = \frac{\cancel{500}}{\cancel{400}}$$

x = 1.25 mL or 1.3 mL Depo-Provera

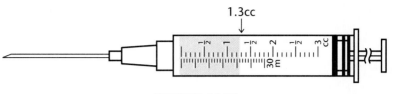

1.3cc

FIGURE 12.72

18. mg:mL = mg:mL

$$100{:}1 = 85{:}x$$

$$\frac{\cancel{100}x}{\cancel{100}} = \frac{85}{100}$$

x = 0.85 mL or 0.9 mL meperidine

mg:mL = mg:mL

$$0.2{:}1 = 0.1{:}x$$

$$\frac{\cancel{0.2}x}{\cancel{0.2}} = \frac{0.1}{0.2}$$

x = 0.5 mL Robinul

0.9 mL + 0.5 mL = 1.4 mL

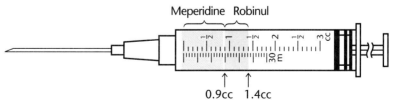

Meperidine   Robinul

0.9cc   1.4cc

FIGURE 12.73

IV

SPECIAL DRUG DOSAGE CALCULATIONS

☆ THE GOAL OF DRUG THERAPY IS TO PRO-duce a therapeutic effect in each patient, yet avoid the adverse reactions and toxic effects that sometimes occur. In order to achieve this goal, you will need to follow special procedures when calculating intravenous infusion rates or when administering drugs to pediatric patients.

In this section, you will learn how to calculate the flow rate, dosage, and infusion time for drugs and solutions administered intravenously. You will also learn two methods for calculating pediatric dosages—one based on body weight, the other on body surface area.

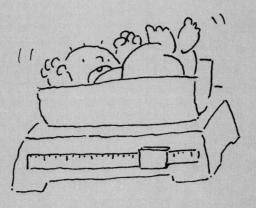

Calculating Intravenous Infusions

13

Objectives

When you finish this chapter, you will be able to:

★ Explain flow rates and drop factors.

★ Calculate the flow rate for continuous intravenous infusions.

★ Calculate the flow rate for intermittent intravenous infusions.

★ Calculate flow rate for intravenous drug dosages.

★ Calculate infusion times.

Chapter Outline

★ Types of Intravenous Infusions

★ Flow Rates and Drop Factors

★ Calculating Flow Rates

★ IVs Ordered at Hourly Rates

★ Microdrip Flow Rates

★ Regulating IV Infusions

★ Calculating Infusion Times

★ Intermittent IV Infusions

★ Infusion Pumps

Introduction

The **intravenous** (IV) route is used to administer fluids, nutrients, electrolytes, blood products, and medications directly into the bloodstream. An increasing number of medications are administered by this route. Continuous IV infusions and intermittent IV infusions are the two most common methods of administering medications intravenously.

Continuous IV infusion administers a medication slowly, over a long period of time, through a primary IV infusion set. **Intermittent IV infusion** introduces a medication at prescribed intervals over a relatively short period of time (30–60 minutes). A medication administered in this fashion is diluted in a small amount of IV solution (50–100 cc). Intermittent IV infusion, sometimes referred to as **IV piggyback (IVPB)**, requires a secondary IV setup that connects to the primary IV tubing.

Types of Intravenous Infusions

---------------------------------- **1** ----------------------------------

bloodstream

Intravenous medications are administered directly into the
_____.

---------------------------------- **2** ----------------------------------

slow
long

Continuous IV infusions administer medications at a
_____ and constant rate over a _____ period
of time. This infusion method provides a relatively constant level
of the drug in the blood.

---------------------------------- **3** ----------------------------------

primary IV infusion set

Continuous IV infusions are administered through a
_____ _____ _____ _____ that
includes a drip chamber to monitor the drip rate, plastic tubing,
and a roller clamp (see Figure 13.1).

---------------------------------- **4** ----------------------------------

4

The roller clamp is used to regulate the rate at which the solution
drips. You measure the flow rate by counting the number of drops
in the drip chamber for 15 seconds and multiplying that number
by _____ to determine the number of drops per minute
(gtt/min).

---------------------------------- **5** ----------------------------------

IV piggyback (IVPB)

Intermittent IV infusions administer medications at prescribed
intervals and are sometimes referred to as _____.

---------------------------------- **6** ----------------------------------

50–100 mL
30–60 minutes

In IVPB infusions the drug is diluted in a small amount of solution
(_____) and infused over a short period of time
(_____).

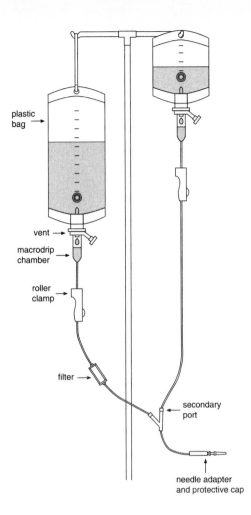

plastic
bag

vent

macrodrip
chamber

roller
clamp

filter

secondary
port

needle adapter
and protective cap

a. Primary IV infusion set   b. Secondary IV infusion set (IVPB)

FIGURE 13.1

7

A _____ _____ _____ that infuses
into the primary IV tubing is used to deliver IVPB medications.

secondary infusion set

DID YOU NOTICE?

The secondary infusion set is hung higher than the primary infusion set. This height difference assists in the gravity flow of IVPB solutions.

8

sterile

As with all parenteral medications and equipment, IV equipment, medications, and solutions must be kept _____.

Flow Rates and Drop Factors

9

gtt/min

When an intravenous solution or medication is needed, the physician orders the type of solution, rate of flow, and the amount of IV solution or medication to be administered over a specific period of time. Ideally the **flow rate** is ordered in **drops per minute** (_____).

10

1000 mL/8h

However, frequently, the order is written in **milliliters per hour (mL/h)**. Consider the order, "1000 mL D5NS IV q.8h." The flow rate is ordered in milliliters per hour or _____.

11

mL/h

When the flow rate is ordered in milliliters per hour (_____), you must convert this flow rate to drops per minute to regulate the flow of the IV solution. To do this, you must know the drop factor and the amount of fluid to be administered over a specified number of hours.

12

smaller
greater

The **drop factor** is the number of drops in one milliliter (gtt/mL) of IV solution. Drop factor depends on the size of the opening in the drip chamber of the IV tubing and varies from one manufacturer to another. The bigger the opening, the larger the drop, and the fewer the number of drops in 1 mL of IV solution. The smaller the opening, the _____ the drop, and the _____ the number of drops in 1 mL of solution.

---------- **13** ----------

The drop factor, abbreviated _____, is printed on the IV infusion set packaging.

gtt/mL

---------- **14** ----------

IV infusion sets that produce large drops per milliliter are called **macrodrip** sets or standard sets and have a drop factor of 10–20 gtt/mL. Infusion sets that produce a drop factor of 60 gtt/mL are called **microdrip** sets (see Table 13.1). The number of drops an IV set delivers in one milliliter is called the _____ _____. Table 13.1 shows the different drop factors.

drop factor

TABLE 13.1 **Common IV Drop Factors**

Infusion Sets	Drop Factors
macrodrip	10 gtt/mL
	15 gtt/mL
	20 gtt/mL
microdrip	60 gtt/mL

---------- **15** ----------

IV infusion sets with drop factors of 10, 15, and 20 gtt/mL are called _____. These sets usually are used for routine adult IV administration (see Figure 13.2).

macrodrips

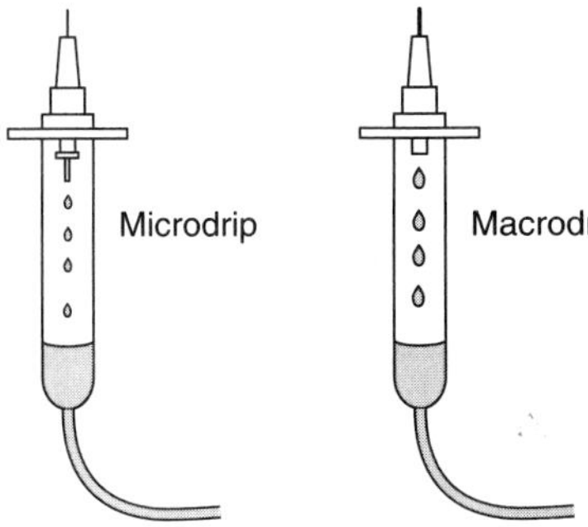

Microdrip   Macrodrip

FIGURE 13.2

---------- **16** ----------

Microdrip infusion sets have a drop factor of _____. They are used to infuse small amounts of solution over a long

60 gtt/mL

time. Microdrip sets also are used when more exact measurements of fluids or drugs are required, such as with pediatric or critically ill patients.

17
---

drop factor

In the clinical setting, you will choose the infusion set based on the amount and type of solution to infuse, the length of infusion time, and the type of patient. Read the IV infusion set packaging to determine the _____ _____. In this book, the drop factor will be given to you for the problems requiring calculations.

Calculating Flow Rates

18
---

gtt/min

When the physician orders IV solutions in milliliters per hour (mL/h), you need to compute the number of drops per minute (_____) to implement the order. This is done by converting the flow rate to milliliters per minute (mL/min) and multiplying by the drop factor.

19

To do this, use a formula that contains 3 factors. The first factor is the rate in mL/h as ordered by the physician. The second is a conversion factor (1 h/60 min) that converts milliliters per hour to milliliters per minute. The third is the drop factor (gtt/mL). Multiplying these three factors together gives you the formula for the flow rate in drops per minute (gtt/min):

$$\frac{mL}{h} \times \frac{1\ h}{60\ min} \times \frac{gtt}{mL} = \frac{gtt}{min}$$

After writing the formula, substitute the numeric values. Then cancel numbers and units and solve for the unknown quantity, x = gtt/min.

For example, let's determine the rate of flow in drops per minute for the order, "1000 mL D5NS IV q8h" (1000 mL in 8 hours). The IV infusion set's drop factor is 15 gtt/mL.

$$\frac{mL}{h} \times \frac{1 \text{ h}}{60 \text{ min}} \times \frac{gtt}{mL} = \frac{gtt}{min} \qquad \leftarrow \text{ formula}$$

$$\frac{1000 \text{ mL}}{8 \text{ h}} \times \frac{1 \text{ h}}{60 \text{ min}} \times \frac{15 \text{ gtt}}{1 \text{ mL}} = x \qquad \leftarrow \text{ numeric value}$$

$$\overset{125}{\underset{1}{\frac{\cancel{1000 \text{ mL}}}{\cancel{8 \text{ h}}}}} \times \underset{4}{\frac{1 \cancel{h}}{\cancel{60} \text{ min}}} \times \overset{1}{\frac{\cancel{15} \text{ gtt}}{1 \cancel{\text{ mL}}}} = x \qquad \leftarrow \text{ cancel}$$

$$\frac{125 \text{ gtt}}{4 \text{ min}} = x$$

You will regulate the IV at _____ to administer 1,000 mL over an 8-hour period of time.

31.25 gtt/min

 REMEMBER

You will use the roller clamp to adjust the rate of flow of IV solutions.

20

The drops per minute calculation is always rounded to the nearest whole number. The rate of flow in the previous example is _____.

31 gtt/min

21

Let's try another example. The physician writes the order, "K.V.O. with 500 mL D5W IV q.12h." The IV infusion set's drop factor is 20 gtt/mL. The flow rate in gtt/min is _____.

$$\frac{mL}{h} \times \frac{1 \text{ h}}{60 \text{ min}}$$

$$\times \frac{gtt}{mL} = \frac{gtt}{min}$$

$$\frac{500 \text{ mL}}{12 \text{ h}} \times \frac{1 \text{ h}}{60 \text{ min}}$$

$$\times \frac{20 \text{ gtt}}{1 \text{ mL}} = x$$

$$\overset{125}{\underset{3}{\frac{\cancel{500 \text{ mL}}}{\cancel{12 \text{ h}}}}} \times \underset{3}{\frac{1 \cancel{h}}{\cancel{60} \text{ min}}}$$

$$\times \overset{1}{\frac{\cancel{20} \text{ gtt}}{1 \cancel{\text{ mL}}}} = x$$

$$x = \frac{125 \text{ gtt}}{9 \text{ min}}$$

$$x = 14 \text{ gtt/min}$$

14 gtt min

a. $\dfrac{\overset{125}{\cancel{500}\,\cancel{mL}}}{\underset{1}{\cancel{4}\,\cancel{hr}}} \times \dfrac{1\,\cancel{hr}}{\underset{6}{\cancel{60}\,min}}$

$\times \dfrac{\overset{1}{\cancel{10}\,gtt}}{1\,\cancel{mL}} = x$

$\qquad x = \dfrac{125\,gtt}{6\,min}$

$\qquad x = 21\,gtt/min$

21 gtt/min

b. $\dfrac{\overset{500}{\cancel{1000}\,\cancel{mL}}}{\underset{3}{\cancel{6}\,\cancel{hr}}} \times \dfrac{1\,\cancel{hr}}{\underset{4}{\cancel{60}\,min}}$

$\times \dfrac{\overset{1}{\cancel{15}\,gtt}}{1\,\cancel{mL}} = x$

$\qquad x = \dfrac{500\,gtt}{12\,min}$

$\qquad x = 42\,gtt/min$

42 gtt/min

c. $\dfrac{\overset{125}{\cancel{1000}\,\cancel{mL}}}{\underset{1}{\cancel{8}\,\cancel{hr}}} \times \dfrac{1\,\cancel{hr}}{\underset{3}{\cancel{60}\,min}}$

$\times \dfrac{\overset{1}{\cancel{20}\,gtt}}{1\,\cancel{mL}} = x$

$\qquad x = \dfrac{125\,gtt}{3\,min}$

$\qquad x = 42\,gtt/min$

42 gtt/min

d. $\dfrac{\overset{125}{\cancel{250}\,\cancel{mL}}}{\underset{4}{\cancel{8}\,\cancel{hr}}} \times \dfrac{1\,\cancel{hr}}{\underset{1}{\cancel{60}\,min}}$

$\times \dfrac{\overset{1}{\cancel{60}\,gtt}}{1\,\cancel{mL}} = x$

$\qquad x = \dfrac{125\,gtt}{4\,min}$

$\qquad x = 31\,gtt/min$

31 gtt/min

— 22 —

Now You Try It

Calculate the flow rate in gtt/min using the following orders and drop factors.

a. The order reads: D5 0.45NS 500 mL IV, infuse in 4 hours. The drop factor is 10 gtt/mL. The flow rate is _____.

b. The order reads: 1000 mL D5W IV q.6h. The drop factor is 15 gtt/mL. The flow rate is _____.

c. The order reads: 1000 mL Ringer's Lactate IV, infuse from 6 a.m. to 2 p.m. The drop factor is 20 gtt/mL. The flow rate is _____.

d. The order reads: 250 mL D5W IV q.8h. The drop factor is 60 gtt/mL. The flow rate is _____.

REMEMBER

Round calculations for drops per minute to the nearest whole number. See Chapter 3, frames 9 through 12, for a review of rounding numbers.

IVs Ordered at Hourly Rates.

---------- **23** ----------

The physician may write IV orders to infuse at an hourly rate of milliliters. For example:

1000 mL D5W IV, infuse @ 100 mL/h.

The hourly rate of infusion is _____. 100 mL/h

---------- **24** ----------

To calculate the rate of flow in gtt/min, use the same formula, but combine the first two fractions by cancelling the hours.

$$\frac{mL}{h} \times \frac{1\ h}{60\ min} \times \frac{gtt}{mL} = \frac{gtt}{min}$$

Use the formula

$$\frac{mL}{60\ min} \times \frac{gtt}{mL} = \frac{gtt}{min}$$

---------- **25** ----------

Consider the order, "1000 mL D5W IV, infuse @ 100 mL/h," again. Let's calculate the flow rate in drops per minute using an IV infusion set with a drop factor of 15 gtt/min.

$$\frac{mL}{60\ min} \times \frac{gtt}{mL} = \frac{gtt}{min} \qquad \longleftarrow \text{ formula}$$

$$\frac{100\ mL}{60\ min} \times \frac{15\ gtt}{1\ mL} = x \qquad \longleftarrow \text{ numeric value}$$

(continues)

$$\frac{25}{\cancel{100}\,\cancel{mL}} \times \frac{\overset{1}{\cancel{15}}\,gtt}{1\,\cancel{mL}} = x \qquad \longleftarrow \text{ cancel}$$
$$\underset{1}{\cancel{4}}$$

$$\frac{25\,gtt}{min} = x$$

25 gtt/min

You will regulate the infusion at _____ .

_____ **26** _____

Now You Try It

Calculate the flow rate in gtt/min when given an hourly IV infusion rate and the drop factor.

a. The order reads: Ringer's Lactate 500 mL infuse @ 75 mL/h. The drop factor is 10 gtt/mL. The flow rate is _____ .

a. $\dfrac{75\,mL}{60\,min} \times \dfrac{10\,gtt}{1\,mL}$
$= x$

$\dfrac{\overset{25}{\cancel{75}}\,\cancel{mL}}{\underset{\cancel{6}}{\cancel{60}}\,min} \times \dfrac{\overset{}{\cancel{10}}\,gtt}{1\,\cancel{mL}}$
$\underset{2}{}$
$= x$

$x = \dfrac{25\,gtt}{2\,min}$

$x = 12.5$ gtt/min

13 gtt/min

b. $\dfrac{25\,mL}{60\,min} \times \dfrac{60\,gtt}{1\,mL}$
$= x$

$\dfrac{25\,\cancel{mL}}{\cancel{60}\,min} \times \dfrac{\cancel{60}\,gtt}{1\,\cancel{mL}}$
$= x$

$x = 25$ gtt/min

25 gtt/min

b. The order reads: D5 $\frac{1}{2}$NS infuse @ 25 mL/h. The drop factor is 60 gtt/mL. The flow rate is _____ .

REMEMBER

You will check the rate of flow of IV solutions by counting the number of drips in 15 seconds and then multiplying that number by 4 to determine the number of drops in a minute (gtt/min).

Microdrip Flow Rates

_____ **27** _____

When infusing medications with a microdrip set, those with a drop factor of _____ , there is a simple method that can

60 gtt/mL

be used to calculate flow rate in gtt/min. Just remember that gtt/min = mL/h.

28

For instance, consider the IV order, "100 mL D5W IV, to infuse at 25 mL/h." The infusion set's drop factor is 60 gtt/mL. The calculated gtt/min is:

$$\frac{25 \text{ mL}}{60 \text{ min}} \times \frac{60 \text{ gtt}}{1 \text{ mL}} = \underline{\hspace{2cm}}$$

25 gtt/min

Note that the flow rate of 25 mL/h is equal to 25 gtt/min. This is because the 60 minutes per hour and the 60 drops per minute cancel each other.

 DID YOU NOTICE?

The infusion time for IV solutions usually does not exceed 24 hours. Whole blood is usually infused in 4 hours.

29

Now look at the order,"D5W 100 mL, infuse @ 35 mL/h." The infusion set's drop factor is 60 gtt/min. The flow rate in gtt/min is _____. Therefore, the flow rate of 35 mL/h is regulated at 35 gtt/min when the drop factor is 60 gtt/min.

$$\frac{\text{mL}}{60 \text{ min}} \times \frac{\text{gtt}}{1 \text{ mL}}$$
$$= \frac{\text{gtt}}{\text{min}}$$
$$\frac{35 \text{ mL}}{60 \text{ min}} \times \frac{60 \text{ gtt}}{1 \text{ mL}}$$
$$= x$$
$$x = 35 \text{ gtt/min}$$

 REMEMBER

The first 2 factors from the formula used to determine flow rates are combined when the infusion time is 60 minutes or less.

30

This simplified method to calculate gtt/min can only be used with a _____ IV infusion set with a drop factor of _____.

microdrip
60 gtt/mL

Regulating IV Infusions

31

Intravenous infusions must be monitored frequently, at least once an hour. Occasionally, IVs will infuse ahead of or behind schedule, requiring recalculation of the flow rate to complete the infusion _____. The remaining amount of IV solution and remaining infusion time are used to obtain the new flow rate in gtt/min.

on time

32

To illustrate how to recalculate an IV flow rate, consider the IV order 500 mL IV, to infuse in 6 hours. The IV infusion set's drop factor is 15 gtt/mL. You will regulate the IV infusion at _____.

$$\frac{500 \text{ mL}}{6} \times \frac{1 \text{h}}{60 \text{ min}}$$

$$\times \frac{15 \text{ gtt}}{1 \text{ mL}} = x$$

$$\frac{\overset{125}{\cancel{500 \text{ mL}}}}{6\,\cancel{h}} \times \frac{1\,\cancel{h}}{\underset{\underset{1}{\cancel{\cancel{A}}}}{\cancel{60}\,\text{min}}}$$

$$\times \frac{\overset{1}{\cancel{15}} \text{ gtt}}{1\,\cancel{\text{mL}}} = x$$

$$x = \frac{125 \text{ gtt}}{6 \text{ min}}$$

$$x = 21 \text{ gtt/min}$$

33

After 3 hours of infusion, 300 mL of solution remains in the IV bag. To complete the infusion of 500 mL D5W in a total of 6 hours, the flow rate must be adjusted so that the remaining _____ of IV solution will infuse in the 3 hours left.

300 mL

34

Do this by calculating a new flow rate. Use the amount of solution left to infuse and the time remaining to determine the value of mL/h. The new value for mL/h is _____.

300 mL/3 h

35

Let's calculate the new flow rate for the above problem:

$$\frac{\text{mL}}{\text{h}} \times \frac{\text{h}}{60 \text{ min}} \times \frac{\text{gtt}}{\text{mL}} = \frac{\text{gtt}}{\text{min}} \qquad \longleftarrow \text{ formula}$$

$$\frac{300 \text{ mL}}{3 \text{ h}} \times \frac{1 \text{ h}}{60 \text{ min}} \times \frac{15 \text{ gtt}}{1 \text{ mL}} = x \qquad \longleftarrow \text{ numeric value}$$

$$\frac{\overset{100}{\cancel{300 \text{ mL}}}}{\underset{1}{\cancel{3 \text{ h}}}} \times \frac{1 \cancel{\text{ h}}}{\underset{4}{\cancel{60} \text{ min}}} \times \frac{\overset{1}{\cancel{15} \text{ gtt}}}{1 \cancel{\text{ mL}}} = x \qquad \longleftarrow \text{ cancel}$$

$$\frac{100 \text{ gtt}}{4 \text{ min}} = x$$

$$\underline{\hspace{2cm}} = x \qquad\qquad\qquad 25 \text{ gtt/min}$$

36

Therefore, the IV infusion flow rate is increased from _____
to _____ gtt/min.

21
25

37

Now You Try It

Calculate the flow rate in gtt/min for each IV order below. Then
calculate the new flow rate in gtt/min based on the information
provided.

a. The order reads: 1000 mL Ringer's Lactate, to infuse over 8
h. The infusion set's drop factor is 20 gtt/mL. You will regulate
the IV infusion at _____.

a. $\dfrac{\overset{125}{\cancel{1000 \text{ mL}}}}{\underset{1}{\cancel{8 \text{ h}}}} \times \dfrac{1 \cancel{\text{ h}}}{\underset{3}{\cancel{60} \text{ min}}}$

$\times \dfrac{\overset{1}{\cancel{20} \text{ gtt}}}{1 \cancel{\text{ mL}}} = x$

$x = \dfrac{125 \text{ gtt}}{3 \text{ min}}$

$x = 42 \text{ gtt/min}$

42 gtt/min

After 5 hours of infusion, 450 mL remains. To complete the
infusion of 1000 mL in a total of 8 hours, the flow rate must
be adjusted. The new flow rate in gtt/min needed to complete
the infusion on time is _____.

$\dfrac{\overset{50}{\underset{1}{\cancel{\overset{150}{\cancel{450 \text{ mL}}}}}}}{\underset{1}{\cancel{3 \text{ h}}}} \times \dfrac{1 \cancel{\text{ h}}}{\underset{3}{\cancel{60} \text{ min}}}$

$\times \dfrac{\overset{1}{\cancel{20} \text{ gtt}}}{1 \cancel{\text{ mL}}} = x$

$x = 50 \text{ gtt/min}$

50 gtt/min

The IV flow rate is adjusted from _____ gtt/min
to _____ gtt/min.

42 gtt/min
50 gtt/min

b. $\dfrac{\overset{125}{\cancel{250}}}{\underset{3}{\cancel{1000\,mL}}} \times \dfrac{1\,\cancel{h}}{\underset{\underset{2}{\cancel{A}}}{\cancel{60}\,min}}$

$\times \dfrac{\overset{1}{\cancel{15}\,gtt}}{1\,\cancel{mL}} = x$

$x = \dfrac{125\,gtt}{6\,min}$

$x = 21\,gtt/min$

21 gtt/min

$\dfrac{\overset{35}{\cancel{70}}}{\underset{\cancel{5}\,\cancel{h}}{\cancel{350\,mL}}} \times \dfrac{1\,\cancel{h}}{\underset{\underset{2}{\cancel{A}}}{\cancel{60}\,min}}$

$\times \dfrac{\overset{1}{\cancel{15}\,gtt}}{1\,\cancel{mL}} = x$

$x = \dfrac{35\,gtt}{2\,min}$

$x = 18\,gtt/min$

18 gtt/min

21 gtt/min
18 gtt/min

8 hours

2 p.m.

b. The order reads: 1000 mL D5NS IV q.12h. The IV infusion set's drop factor is 15 gtt/mL. You will regulate the IV infusion at _____.

After 7 hours of infusion, 350 mL remain. To complete the infusion of 1000 mL D5NS in a total of 12 h, the flow rate must be adjusted. The new flow rate in gtt/min needed to complete the infusion on time is _____.

The IV flow rate is adjusted from _____ gtt/min to _____ gtt/min.

Calculating Infusion Times

38

Occasionally, it may become important to calculate the total infusion time for an IV. Knowledge of infusion time is helpful in determining when certain laboratory tests are scheduled or when the next IV solution needs to be prepared. In the order, "D5W 1000 mL IV q.8h," the infusion time for 1000 mL D5W is _____.

39

If 1000 mL D5W infusion is started at 6 a.m., it will be completed at _____.

40

To calculate the infusion, the amount to be infused is divided by the rate. In the order, "D5 $\frac{1}{4}$NS 500 mL IV @ 50 mL/h," divide the total volume by mL/h. For example:

$$500 \text{ mL} \div \frac{50 \text{ mL}}{1 \text{ h}} = \text{infusion time}$$

When solved, the infusion time is _____.

REMEMBER

The divisor, mL/h, must be inverted before the problem can be solved.

$$500 \text{ mL} \div \frac{50 \text{ mL}}{1 \text{ h}}$$
$$= x$$
$$\frac{\overset{10}{\cancel{500 \text{ mL}}}}{1} \times \frac{1 \text{ h}}{\cancel{50 \text{ mL}}}$$
$$= x$$
$$x = 10 \text{ hours}$$

41

For the order, "D5W 1000 mL @ 75 mL/h," the infusion time is _____.

$$1000 \text{ mL} \div \frac{75 \text{ mL}}{1 \text{ h}}$$
$$= x$$
$$\frac{1000 \text{ mL}}{1} \times \frac{1 \text{ h}}{75 \text{ mL}}$$
$$= x$$
$$x = 13.3 \text{ hours}$$

42

To convert 0.3 hours to minutes, simply multiply by 60 minutes. Therefore 0.3 × 60 = 18. The infusion time for 1,000 mL D5W @ 75 mL/h is _____ hours and _____ minutes.

13   18

43

Now You Try It

Using the given IV orders, calculate the infusion times.

a. The order reads: D5W 500 mL @ 20 mL/h. The IV will infuse in _____.

a. $$500 \text{ mL} \div \frac{20 \text{ mL}}{1 \text{ h}}$$
$$= x$$
$$\frac{\overset{25}{\cancel{500 \text{ mL}}}}{1} \times \frac{1 \text{ h}}{\underset{1}{\cancel{20 \text{ mL}}}}$$
$$= x$$
$$x = 25 \text{ hours}$$

b. 500 mL ÷ $\dfrac{25\ mL}{1\ h}$

    = x

$$\dfrac{\overset{20}{\cancel{500\ mL}}}{1} \times \dfrac{1\ h}{\underset{1}{\cancel{25\ mL}}}$$

    = x

x = 20 hours; 2 a.m.

---

c. 1000 mL ÷ $\dfrac{150\ mL}{1\ h}$

    = x

$$\dfrac{\overset{20}{\cancel{1000\ mL}}}{1} \times \dfrac{1\ h}{\underset{3}{\cancel{150\ mL}}}$$

    = x

x = 6.7 hours

6 hours & 42 min.
  = 10:42 p.m.

---

d. 500 mL ÷ $\dfrac{125\ mL}{1\ h}$

    = x

$$\dfrac{\overset{4}{\cancel{500\ mL}}}{1} \times \dfrac{1\ h}{\underset{1}{\cancel{125\ mL}}}$$

    = x

x = 4 hours

IV Piggyback
IVPB

---

50   100

---

b. The order reads: D5NS 500 mL @ 25 mL/h. If the IV is started at 6 a.m., it will be completed by _____.

c. The order reads: D5RL 1000 mL @ 150 mL/h. If the IV is started at 4 p.m., it will be completed by _____.

d. The order reads: 500 mL whole blood @ 125 mL/h. The IV will infuse in _____.

Intermittent IV Infusions

—————————————— **44** ——————————————

Medications administered as intermittent IV infusions are referred to as _____ _____, abbreviated as _____.

—————————————— **45** ——————————————

Medications are diluted in _____ to _____ milliliters of IV solution and infused in 60 minutes or less. Drug package inserts or drug references provide the guidelines for dilution amounts and infusion time if the physician's order does not include this information.

―――――――――――― **46** ――――――――――――

To calculate infusion times for one hour or less, remember to use the formula,

$$\frac{mL}{min} \times \frac{gtt}{mL} = \frac{gtt}{min}$$

―――――――――――― **47** ――――――――――――

Let's determine the infusion rate in drops per minute for the order, "Cimetidine 300 mg in 100 mL D5W IVPB to infuse over 30 minutes q.6h." The IVPB infusion set's drop factor is 10 gtt/mL.

$$\frac{mL}{min} \times \frac{gtt}{mL} = \frac{gtt}{min}$$

$$\frac{100 \text{ mL}}{30 \text{ min}} \times \frac{10 \text{ gtt}}{1 \text{ mL}} = x$$

$$\frac{100 \text{ mL}}{3 \text{ min}} \times \frac{10 \text{ gtt}}{1 \text{ mL}} = x$$

$$\frac{100 \text{ gtt}}{3 \text{ min}} = x$$

$$\text{_____} = x$$

You will regulate the IVPB infusion at _____.

$\dfrac{33.3 \text{ gtt}}{min}$ or $\dfrac{33 \text{ gtt}}{min}$
33 gtt/min

―――――――――――― **48** ――――――――――――

Now You Try It

Calculate the flow rate for the following IVPB using the given IV orders and drop factors.

a. The order reads: Kefzol 1 g IVPB q.6h. Kefzol is mixed in 50 mL D5W and infused over 20 minutes. The drop factor is 20 gtt/mL. You will regulate the IVPB at _____.

a. $\dfrac{50 \text{ mL}}{20 \text{ min}} \times \dfrac{20 \text{ gtt}}{1 \text{ mL}}$
$= x$
$x = 50 \text{ gtt/min}$
50 gtt/min

b. $\dfrac{100\ \cancel{mL}}{\underset{3}{\cancel{45}}\ min} \times \dfrac{\cancel{15}\ gtt}{1\ \cancel{mL}}$

$\qquad = x$

$x = \dfrac{100\ gtt}{3\ min}$

$x = 33\ gtt/min$

33 gtt/min

U/h
mL/h

1000 mL/20,000 U

b. The order reads: clindamycin 600 mg IVPB q.8h. Infuse 600 mg/100 mL D5W over 45 minutes. The drop factor is 15 gtt/mL. You will regulate the IVPB at _____.

DID YOU NOTICE?

When calculating the flow rate in gtt/min using a micro-drip infusion set, the 60 gtt and 60 min cancel each other out.

$$\dfrac{25\ mL}{60\ min} \times \dfrac{60\ gtt}{1\ mL} = 25\ gtt/min$$

Infusion Pumps

49

Some IV infusions are administered by an **electronic infusion pump** to insure accuracy. IV medications such as pitocin, insulin, and heparin, which are ordered in units, are also administered by an electronic IV infusion pump. In these situations, the ordered IV infusion or ordered dosage of medication such as units/hour (_____) must be converted to milliliters per hour (_____) to calculate the flow rate used to set the electronic IV infusion pump.

50

To accomplish this, multiply the dosage order (U/h) by the dosage strength (mL/U). For example:

$$\dfrac{U}{h} \times \dfrac{mL}{U} = \dfrac{mL}{h}$$

Consider the order, "heparin 800 U/h." The available IV solution is D5W 1000 mL with heparin 20,000 U, with a dosage strength of _____.

51

To calculate the flow rate in mL/h, the setup looks like

$$\frac{800 \text{ U}}{1 \text{ h}} \times \frac{1000 \text{ mL}}{20,000 \text{ U}} = \text{mL/h}$$

The flow rate in mL/h is _____. The electronic infusion pump is set at _____.

$$\frac{\overset{40}{\cancel{800} \text{ U}}}{1 \text{ h}} \times \frac{\overset{1}{\cancel{1000} \text{ mL}}}{\underset{1}{\cancel{20,000} \text{ U}}}$$
$$= x$$
$$x = 40 \text{ mL/h}$$
40 mL per hour

──────────── **52** ────────────

For the order, "Add 100 U regular insulin to 500 mL IV solution and administer at 8 U/h," the dosage strength is _____.

500 mL/100 U

──────────── **53** ────────────

The flow rate in mL/h for insulin is _____. The electronic infusion pump is set at _____.

$$\frac{8 \text{ U}}{1 \text{ h}} \times \frac{\cancel{500} \text{ mL}}{\cancel{100} \text{ U}} = x$$
$$x = 40 \text{ mL/h}$$
40 mL per hour

──────────── **54** ────────────

For the order, "Add 10 U pitocin to 1000 mL D5W and administer 600 mU/h of pitocin," the dosage strength is _____.

1000 mL/10 U

──────────── **55** ────────────

When the available solution and requested dosage are in different units of measurement, an appropriate equivalent fraction must be used. The equivalent fraction in this case is 1 unit (U)/1000 milliunits (mU) or 1 U/1000 mU. To change 600 mU to mL/h the setup is:

$$\frac{\text{mU}}{\text{h}} \times \frac{1 \text{ U}}{1000 \text{ mU}} \times \text{_____} = \text{mL/h}$$

mL/U

──────────── **56** ────────────

To calculate mL/h for pitocin, the problem setup is:

$$\frac{600 \text{ mU}}{1 \text{ h}} \times \frac{1 \text{ U}}{1000 \text{ mU}} \times \frac{1000 \text{ mL}}{10 \text{ U}} = x$$

The flow rate in mL/h is _____. The electronic infusion pump is set at _____.

$x = 60 \text{ mL/h}$
60 mL per hour

57
---

60 gtt/min

If a microdrip infusion set is used rather than an infusion pump, the flow rate for pitocin is _____.

REMEMBER

When the drop factor is 60 gtt/min (microdrip infusion set), the mL/h = gtt/min.

58

Now You Try It

Calculate the rate of flow you will set the infusion pumps at using the following IV orders.

a.
$$\text{a.} \quad \frac{\cancel{1000}\,\cancel{U}}{1\text{ h}} \times \frac{\overset{20}{\cancel{500}}\text{ mL}}{\underset{1}{\cancel{25000}\,\cancel{U}}}$$
$$= x$$
$$x = 20\text{ mL/h}$$
20 mL/h

a. The order reads: Add 25,000 U of heparin to 500 mL D5W. Administer @ 1000 U/h. You will set the infusion pump at _____.

b.
$$\text{b.} \quad \frac{\cancel{10}\,\cancel{U}}{1\text{ h}} \times \frac{\cancel{250}\text{ mL}}{\cancel{100}\,\cancel{U}}$$
$$= x$$
$$x = 25\text{ mL/h}$$
25 mL/h

b. The order reads: Add 100 U regular insulin to 250 mL 0.9% NS, then administer 10 U/h of regular insulin. You will set the infusion pump at _____.

c.
$$\text{c.} \quad \frac{\overset{50}{\cancel{500}\,m\cancel{U}}}{1\text{ h}} \times \frac{\overset{1}{\cancel{500}}\text{ mL}}{\underset{\underset{1}{10}}{\cancel{5000}\,m\cancel{U}}}$$
$$= x$$
$$x = 50\text{ mL/h}$$
50 mL/h

c. The order reads: Add 5000 mU pitocin to 500 mL D5W. Administer @ 500 mU/h. You will set the infusion pump at _____.

d.
$$\text{d.} \quad \frac{\cancel{750}\,m\cancel{U}}{1\text{ h}} \times \frac{1\,\cancel{U}}{\cancel{1000}\,m\cancel{U}}$$
$$\times \frac{\cancel{750}\text{ mL}}{\cancel{10}\,\cancel{U}}$$
$$= x$$
$$x = \frac{5625\text{ mL}}{100\text{ h}}$$
$$x = 56\text{ mL/h}$$
56 mL/h

d. The order reads: Add pitocin 10 U to 750 mL D5W. Administer @ 750 mU/h. You will set the infusion pump at _____.

REMEMBER

1 U = 1000 milliunits

☆ What You've Achieved!

★ You can explain flow rates and drop factors.

★ You can calculate flow rates for continuous and intermittent intravenous infusions.

★ You know how to determine infusion times.

★ You have learned how to calculate flow rates for infusion pumps.

Fantastic! What you've learned in this chapter will help you perform calculations necessary for infusion of IV solutions and medications. Before moving forward, take the review test to determine your mastery of calculations for IV therapy. If you get more than one wrong in section A, C, D, E, and F or two wrong in section B, consider studying that portion of the chapter again.

Review Test

—————————————————— **A** ——————————————————

Complete the following statements.

1. IV medications are administered directly into the _____.

2. Intermittent IV medication infusions are prescribed at _____ intervals and infused over a short period of time ranging from _____ to _____.

3. When administering intermittent IV medications, (abbreviated _____), the drug is diluted in _____ mL of solution.

4. Infusion sets that have a drop factor of 10–20 gtt/min are called _____.

5. Microdrip sets have a drop factor of _____.

B

Calcuate the flow rate in gtt/min using the following IV orders and drop factors.

6. The order reads: D5 $\frac{1}{4}$NS 500 mL/24 h K.V.O. The drop factor is 60 gtt/mL. The flow rate is _____.

7. The order reads: D5W 1500 mL IV 6 a.m. to 6 p.m. The drop factor is 15 gtt/mL. The flow rate is _____.

8. The order reads: 500 mL D5W IV from 8 p.m. to 11 p.m. The drop factor is 10 gtt/mL. The flow rate is _____.

9. The order reads: Hyperalimentation 1100 mL over 12 h. The drop factor is 20 gtt/mL. The flow rate is _____.

10. The order reads: D5 $\frac{1}{2}$NS 1000 mL @ 150 mL/h. The drop factor is 20 gtt/mL. The flow rate is _____.

C

Calculate the flow rate in gtt/min for IVPB infusions using the following orders and drop factors.

11. The order reads: ampicillin 1 g IVPB q.8h. Mix in 50 mL NSS. Infuse over 40 minutes. The drop factor is 20 gtt/mL. The flow rate is _____.

12. The order reads: Cleocin 300 mg IVPB q.6h. Mix in 50 mL D5W. Infuse over 15 minutes. The drop factor is 15 gtt/mL. The flow rate is _____.

13. The order reads: Solu-Medrol 100 mg IVPB q.6h. Mix in 75 mL D5W. Infuse over 25 minutes. The drop factor is 10 gtt/mL. The flow rate is _____.

D

Calculate the new flow rate in gtt/min using the following IV orders, drop factors, and situations.

14. The order reads: D5NS 1000 mL q.8h. At 11 a.m. 400 mL remains. The infusion must be completed at 4 p.m. The drop factor is 15 gtt/mL. The new flow rate is _____.

15. The order reads: 1000 mL NSS IV q.10h. The IV started at 11 a.m. At 4 p.m., 550 mL remains. The drop factor is 20 gtt/min. The new flow rate is _____.

16. The order reads: D5W 1000 mL 7 a.m. to 5 p.m. At 2 p.m., 325 mL remains. The drop factor is 10 gtt/mL. The new flow rate is _____.

---------------------------------- **E** ----------------------------------

Calculate the flow rate in mL/h you will set the infusion pump at using the following IV orders.

17. The order reads: heparin 1500 U in 500 mL NSS to run @ 120 U/h. The flow rate is _____.

18. The order reads: insulin 100 U in 250 mL NSS to infuse @ 7 U/h. The flow rate is _____.

---------------------------------- **F** ----------------------------------

Calculate the infusion times.

19. The order reads: D5 $\frac{1}{4}$ 1000 mL to run @ 80 mL/h. What time will the infusion be completed if it started at 8 a.m.? _____

20. The order reads: NSS 250 mL with regular insulin 100 U to run @ 15 mL/h. How many hours will the infusion last? _____

Answers for Review Test

1. bloodstream   2. specific, 30, 60 minutes   3. IVPB, 50–100 mL

---

4. macrodrip   5. 60 gtt/mL   6. $\dfrac{\overset{125}{\cancel{500}\,\text{mL}}}{\underset{6}{\cancel{24}\,\text{h}}} \times \dfrac{1\,\cancel{h}}{\underset{1}{\cancel{60}\,\text{min}}} \times \dfrac{\overset{1}{\cancel{60}\,\text{gtt}}}{1\,\cancel{\text{mL}}} = 21\ \text{gtt/min}$

---

7. $\dfrac{\overset{125}{\cancel{1500}\,\text{mL}}}{\underset{1}{\cancel{12}\,\text{h}}} \times \dfrac{1\,\cancel{h}}{\underset{4}{\cancel{60}\,\text{min}}} \times \dfrac{\overset{15}{\cancel{15}\,\text{gtt}}}{1\,\cancel{\text{mL}}} = \dfrac{125\ \text{gtt}}{4\ \text{min}} = 31\ \text{gtt/min}$

---

8. $\dfrac{\overset{250}{\cancel{500}\,\text{mL}}}{3\,\cancel{h}} \times \dfrac{1\,\cancel{h}}{\underset{3}{\cancel{60}\,\text{min}}} \times \dfrac{\overset{10}{\cancel{10}\,\text{gtt}}}{1\,\cancel{\text{mL}}} = \dfrac{250\ \text{gtt}}{9\ \text{min}} = 28\ \text{gtt/min}$

---

9. $\dfrac{\overset{275}{\cancel{1100}\,\text{mL}}}{\underset{3}{\cancel{12}\,\text{h}}} \times \dfrac{1\,\cancel{h}}{\underset{3}{\cancel{60}\,\text{min}}} \times \dfrac{\overset{20}{\cancel{20}\,\text{gtt}}}{1\,\cancel{\text{mL}}} = \dfrac{275\ \text{gtt}}{9\ \text{min}} = 31\ \text{gtt/min}$

10.
$$\frac{\overset{50}{\cancel{150}\,\cancel{mL}}}{\underset{1}{\underset{\cancel{3}}{\cancel{60}\,\text{min}}}} \times \frac{\overset{1}{\cancel{20}\,\text{gtt}}}{1\,\cancel{mL}} = 50\ \text{gtt/min}$$

11.
$$\frac{\overset{25}{\cancel{50}\,\cancel{mL}}}{\underset{1}{\underset{\cancel{2}}{\cancel{40}\,\text{min}}}} \times \frac{\overset{1}{\cancel{20}\,\text{gtt}}}{1\,\cancel{mL}} = 25\ \text{gtt/min}$$

12.
$$\frac{50\,\cancel{mL}}{\underset{1}{\cancel{15}\,\text{min}}} \times \frac{\overset{15}{\cancel{15}\,\text{gtt}}}{1\,\cancel{mL}} = 50\ \text{gtt/min}$$

13.
$$\frac{\overset{3}{\cancel{75}\,\cancel{mL}}}{\underset{1}{\cancel{25}\,\text{min}}} \times \frac{10\,\text{gtt}}{1\,\cancel{mL}} = 30\ \text{gtt/min}$$

14.
$$\frac{\overset{\overset{20}{\cancel{100}}}{\cancel{400}\,\cancel{mL}}}{\underset{1}{\cancel{5}\,\cancel{h}}} \times \frac{1\,\cancel{h}}{\underset{\underset{1}{\cancel{4}}}{\cancel{60}\,\text{min}}} \times \frac{\overset{1}{\cancel{15}\,\text{gtt}}}{1\,\cancel{mL}} = 20\ \text{gtt/min}$$

15.
$$\frac{\overset{110}{\cancel{550}\,\cancel{mL}}}{\underset{1}{\cancel{5}\,\cancel{h}}} \times \frac{1\,\cancel{h}}{\underset{3}{\cancel{60}\,\text{min}}} \times \frac{\overset{1}{\cancel{20}\,\text{gtt}}}{1\,\cancel{mL}} = \frac{110\ \text{gtt}}{3\ \text{min}} = 37\ \text{gtt/min}$$

16.
$$\frac{325\,\cancel{mL}}{3\,\cancel{h}} \times \frac{1\,\cancel{h}}{\underset{6}{\cancel{60}\,\text{min}}} \times \frac{\overset{1}{\cancel{10}\,\text{gtt}}}{1\,\cancel{mL}} = \frac{325\ \text{gtt}}{18\ \text{min}} = 18\ \text{gtt/min}$$

17.
$$\frac{\overset{40}{\cancel{120}\,\cancel{U}}}{1\ \text{h}} \times \frac{\overset{500\ \text{mL}}{}}{\underset{1}{\underset{\cancel{3}}{\cancel{1500}\,\cancel{U}}}} = 40\ \text{mL per hour}$$

18.
$$\frac{7\,\cancel{U}}{1\ \text{h}} \times \frac{\overset{2.5}{\cancel{250}\ \text{mL}}}{\underset{1}{\cancel{100}\,\cancel{U}}} = 17.5\ \text{mL} = 18\ \text{mL per hour}$$

19.
$$1000\ \text{mL} \div \frac{80\ \text{mL}}{1\ \text{h}} = \frac{\overset{25}{\cancel{1000}\,\cancel{mL}}}{1} \times \frac{1\ \text{h}}{\underset{2}{\cancel{80}\,\cancel{mL}}} = \frac{25\ \text{h}}{2} = 12.5\ \text{h}$$

$x = 12$ hours, 30 minutes, 8:30 p.m.

20.
$$250\ \text{mL} \div \frac{15\ \text{mL}}{1\ \text{h}} = \frac{\overset{50}{\cancel{250}\,\cancel{mL}}}{1} \times \frac{1\ \text{h}}{\underset{3}{\cancel{15}\,\cancel{mL}}} = \frac{50\ \text{h}}{3} = 16.7\ \text{h} \qquad x = 16\ \text{hours, 42 minutes}$$

Drug Dosages for Pediatric Patients

14

Objectives

When you finish this chapter, you will be able to:

★ Calculate the safe dosage for infants and children according to the body-surface-area and dosage-per-kilogram-of-body-weight methods.

★ Calculate body surface area using a nomogram.

★ Verify safe dosages by comparing the prescribed dosage for the pediatric patient against the recommended dosage.

Chapter Outline

★ Calculating Dosages by Body Weight

★ Converting Pounds to Kilograms

★ Calculating Body Surface Area

★ Calculating Dosages by Body Surface Area

★ Calculating Pediatric Dosages from Adult Dosages

★ Calculating Daily Fluid Needs

Introduction

The body's physiologic maturity significantly affects the way drugs work. For example, because an infant's or child's physiologic processes are not as fully developed as those of an adult, its body will not absorb, distribute, metabolize, or excrete drugs at the same rate as an adult's body. Moreover, a child's body does not need as much medication to reach the same therapeutic level as an adult's body. For these reasons, pediatric drug dosages almost always are less than the recommended adult dosages for the same medications.

You will need to follow special methods in order to safely calculate pediatric drug dosages for **infants** (birth to 12 months) and **children** (one year to 12 years). The two most accurate methods used to check for safe dosage ranges and to calculate pediatric dosages are the dosage-per-kilogram-of-body-weight (mg/kg) method and the body-surface-area (BSA) method.

Calculating Dosages by Body Weight

—————————————— **1** ——————————————

physiologic processes

Infant's and children's _____ _____ are not as fully developed as those of adults.

—————————————— **2** ——————————————

absorbed
distributed
metabolized
excreted

The physiology of children influences how drugs are _____, _____, _____, and _____ by the body.

—————————————— **3** ——————————————

less

Because infants and children have different physiologic processes and smaller bodies than adults, they usually receive _____ medication per dose than adults.

—————————————— **4** ——————————————

dosage range

You will need to follow special procedures when calculating dosages for infants and children in order to determine the safe _____ _____ for prescribed medications. Although the physician prescribes the drug dosage, you are legally responsible for administering a safe amount.

—————————————— **5** ——————————————

dosage-per-kilogram-
of-body-weight
body-surface-area

The two most accurate methods you will use to calculate pediatric drug dosages are _____ _____ _____ _____ _____ _____ and _____ _____ _____. These methods have replaced the use of other formulas such as Clark's, Young's, and Freid's rules (see appendix C).

6

The **dosage-per-kilogram-of-body-weight** (_____)
method is one of the most accurate and the most commonly used
methods for calculating pediatric dosages. You will also use this
method to verify that prescribed dosages fall within the recommended dosage ranges.

mg/kg

7

This method multiplies the specific dose in milligrams, micrograms, or units of the ordered drug by the infant's or child's body
weight in _____.

kilograms

8

Medication labels, drug package inserts, and drug references
provide the **recommended dosage range** in _____,
_____, or _____ per kilogram. Frequently, the
dose is calculated for 24 hours in evenly divided dosages.

milligrams
micrograms
units

9

Use the ratio-and-proportion method to determine the safe
dosage range. To do so, multiply the minimum and maximum
recommended dosages by the infant's or child's weight in
_____.

kilograms

10

Let's review the three steps of the ratio-and-proportion method.
First, select two equal ratios and write them as a proportion
labeled "_____" ratio and "_____ _____
_____" ratio. The recommended dosage becomes the
"known" ratio and the prescribed dosage becomes the "want-to-
know" ratio. Second, write the units in proportion form and then
rewrite using numeric values. Third, multiply the means and
extremes and solve for the unknown quantity.

known
want-to-know

11

Consider a drug order that reads, Keflex 150 mg p.o. q.6h, for a
child weighing 15 kg. Look at Figure 14.1. The recommended

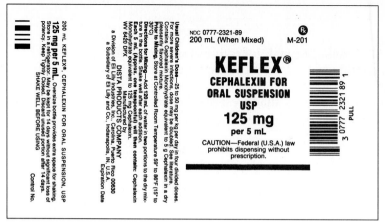

FIGURE 14.1

25 / 50 mg

dosage is _____ to _____ per kg per day in four divided doses.

 DID YOU NOTICE?

You can find the recommended dosage for Keflex under the heading "Usual Children's Dose."

12

Let's determine the minimum dose you would administer using the ratio-and-proportion method.

known = want-to-know

mg:kg = mg:kg ⟵ units in proportional form

25:1 = x:15 ⟵ quantities in proportional form

25:1 = x:15 ⟵ multiply means and extremes

x = 375 mg

The minimum dose of Keflex you would administer in 24 hours

375 mg

is _____.

--------------------------------- **13** ---------------------------------

Now determine the maximum dose you would administer. The maximum dose of Keflex you can administer in 24 hours is _____.

mg:kg = mg:kg

50:1 = x:15

x = 750 mg
750 mg maximum dose

--------------------------------- **14** ---------------------------------

The safe dosage range for Keflex is _____ to _____ per 24 hours.

375 mg
750 mg

--------------------------------- **15** ---------------------------------

You will determine the minimum and maximum individual doses by dividing each range by the number of doses specified per 24 hours. The number of doses of Keflex in 24 hours is _____.

4

--------------------------------- **16** ---------------------------------

The range for the amount of drug permitted for one dose of Keflex is _____ to _____.

375 mg ÷ 4 = 93.75 mg
750 mg ÷ 4 = 187.5 mg
94 mg minimum / 188 mg maximum

--------------------------------- **17** ---------------------------------

The ordered dose of Keflex, 150 mg q.6h, is a _____ dose.

safe

--------------------------------- **18** ---------------------------------

Look at Figure 14.1 again. The amount of Keflex you will administer to provide a 150-mg dose is _____.

mg:mL = mg:mL

125:5 = 150:x

125x = 750
x = 6 mL
6 mL

--------------------------------- **19** ---------------------------------

Remember, you are legally responsible for the patient's safety when administering medications. You must verify that the prescribed dose falls within the range of the recommended dose. If the prescribed dose is too high to be safe or too low to be therapeutic you must not administer the medication, but should consult with the physician who prescribed it. You will only administer those medications that are within the _____ range.

recommended

REMEMBER

★ Calculate the total dosage permitted for the child's or infant's body weight.

★ Compare the result with the physician's order.

★ If the dose falls within the recommended range, calculate and administer the prescribed medication.

★ If the dose is too small or too large, do not give the medication; consult with the prescribing doctor.

20

Now You Try It

Calculate the safe dosage range for 24 hours and the divided dosages using the following drug orders and medication labels. Calculate the amount of medication you will administer.

a. The order reads: Pen-Vee-K 200 mg p.o. q.6h. The child's weight is 25 kilograms. The recommended dose is: 25–50 mg/kg/day in divided doses q.6h. The dosage range is _____ to _____. The divided dosage range is _____ to _____. Is the dose therapeutic and safe? _____ The available dosage is: Pen-Vee-K 250 mg/5 mL. You will administer _____.

a. mg:kg = mg:kg

$25:1 = x:25$

$x = 625$ mg min

$50:1 = x:25$

$x = 1250$ mg max

625 mg / 1250 mg

156.3 mg / 312.5 mg

Yes

mg:mL = mg:mL

$250:5 = 200:x$

$250x = 1000$

$x = 4$ mL

4 mL Pen-Vee-K

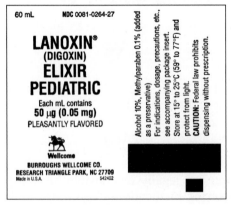

60 mL   NDC 0081-0264-27

LANOXIN®
(DIGOXIN)
ELIXIR
PEDIATRIC

Each mL contains
50 µg (0.05 mg)
PLEASANTLY FLAVORED

Wellcome
BURROUGHS WELLCOME CO.
RESEARCH TRIANGLE PARK, NC 27709
Made in U.S.A.   542402

Alcohol 10%, Methylparaben 0.1% (added as a preservative)
For indications, dosage, precautions, etc., see accompanying package insert.
Store at 15° to 25°C (59° to 77°F) and protect from light.
CAUTION: Federal law prohibits dispensing without prescription.

FIGURE 14.2

b. The order reads: digoxin 45 mcg p.o. b.i.d (see Figure 14.2). The infant's weight is 8 kilograms. The recommended dose is: less than 2 yr, 10–12 mcg/kg/day in divided doses q.12h. The dosage range is _____ to _____. The divided dosage range is _____ to _____. Is the dose therapeutic and safe? _____ You will administer _____.

b. mcg:kg = mcg:kg

$10:1 = x:8$

$x = 80$ mcg min

$12:1 = x:8$

$x = 96$ mcg max

80 mcg / 96 mcg

40 mcg / 48 mcg

Yes

mcg:mL = mcg:mL

$50:1 = 45:x$

$50x = 45$

$x = 0.9$ mL

0.9 mL digoxin

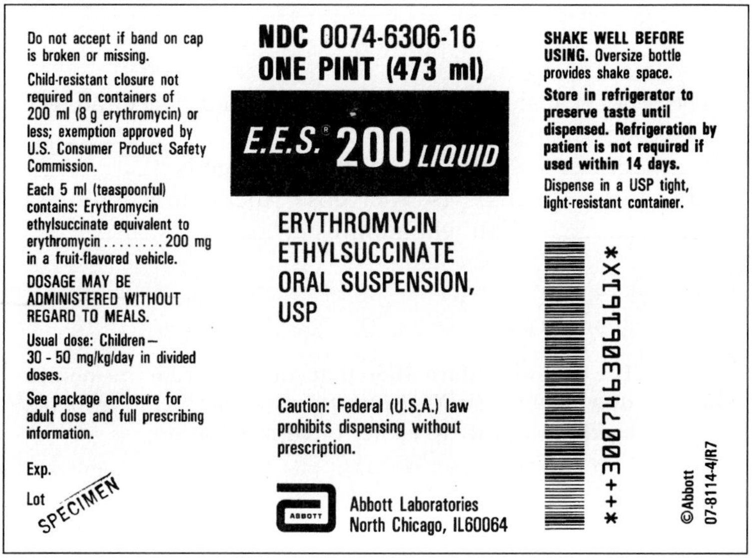

Do not accept if band on cap is broken or missing.	NDC 0074-6306-16	SHAKE WELL BEFORE USING. Oversize bottle provides shake space.

NDC 0074-6306-16
ONE PINT (473 ml)

Do not accept if band on cap is broken or missing.

Child-resistant closure not required on containers of 200 ml (8 g erythromycin) or less; exemption approved by U.S. Consumer Product Safety Commission.

Each 5 ml (teaspoonful) contains: Erythromycin ethylsuccinate equivalent to erythromycin . . . . 200 mg in a fruit-flavored vehicle.

DOSAGE MAY BE ADMINISTERED WITHOUT REGARD TO MEALS.

Usual dose: Children — 30 - 50 mg/kg/day in divided doses.

See package enclosure for adult dose and full prescribing information.

Exp.

Lot

SPECIMEN

E.E.S. **200** LIQUID

ERYTHROMYCIN ETHYLSUCCINATE ORAL SUSPENSION, USP

Caution: Federal (U.S.A.) law prohibits dispensing without prescription.

Abbott Laboratories
North Chicago, IL60064

SHAKE WELL BEFORE USING. Oversize bottle provides shake space.

Store in refrigerator to preserve taste until dispensed. Refrigeration by patient is not required if used within 14 days.

Dispense in a USP tight, light-resistant container.

©Abbott 07-8114-4/R7

FIGURE 14.3

c. The order reads: E.E.S. 150 mg p.o. t.i.d. The child weighs 18 kilograms. The dosage range is _____ to _____. The divided dosage range is _____ to _____. Is the dose therapeutic and safe? _____

c. mg:kg = mg:kg

$30:1 = x:18$

$x = 540$ mg min

$50:1 = x:18$

$x = 900$ mg max

540 mg / 900 mg

180 / 300 mg

No

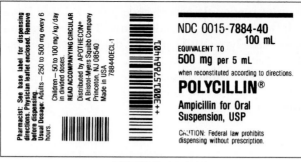

FIGURE 14.4

d. The order reads: Polycillin 400 mg p.o. q.i.d. The child weighs 24 kilograms. The dosage range is _____ to _____. The divided dosage range is _____ to _____. Is the dose therapeutic and safe? _____ You will administer _____.

> **REMEMBER**
>
> The essential information that you need from the medication label (or package insert) is the dosage range in mg/kg/day and the frequency of administration.

Converting Pounds to Kilograms

21

Many hospitals record body weight in pounds. If an infant's or child's weight is expressed in pounds, it must be converted to _____ before determining a safe pediatric drug dosage range.

22

You will use the ratio-and-proportion method to convert pounds to kilograms. Use the equivalent, 2.2 lbs = 1 kg. For example, 35 pounds is equivalent to _____.

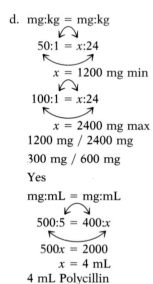

d. mg:kg = mg:kg

    50:1 = x:24

      x = 1200 mg min

100:1 = x:24

      x = 2400 mg max

1200 mg / 2400 mg

300 mg / 600 mg

Yes

mg:mL = mg:mL

  500:5 = 400:x

  500x = 2000

     x = 4 mL

4 mL Polycillin

kilograms

lbs:kg = lbs:kg

  2.2:1 = 35:x

  2.2:1 = 35:x

2.2x = 35

  x = 15.9 kg

15.9 kilograms

REMEMBER

If an infant's or child's weight is expressed in pounds, it must be converted to kilograms before determining a safe pediatric dose range. If you need a review of converting pounds to kilograms, see Chapter 8.

23

Now You Try It

Convert the following pounds to kilograms. Round your answers to the nearest tenth.

a. 6 lbs 8 oz   = _____ kg

b. 14 lbs   = _____ kg

c. 56 lbs   = _____ kg

d. 21 lbs 8 oz = _____ kg

e. 45 lbs   = _____ kg

DID YOU NOTICE?

If the infant's or child's weight is in pounds and ounces, you must convert the ounces to pounds before converting the weight to kilograms. For example, 6 lbs 8 oz is equivalent to 6.5 lbs (1 lb = 16 oz).

Calculating Body Surface Area

24

The second method of calculating pediatric dosages and dosage ranges is the _____ _____ _____ (**BSA**) method. This method uses a nomogram, shown on the inside back cover, to convert a child's height and weight into body surface area in **square meters** (M^2).

---

a. lb:kg = lb:kg
   2.2:1 = 6.5:x
   $2.2x = 6.5$
   $x = 2.95$ or 3 kg

b. lb:kg = lb:kg
   2.2:1 = 14:x
   $2.2x = 14$
   $x = 6.36$ or 6.4 kg

c. lb:kg = lb:kg
   2.2:1 = 56:x
   $2.2x = 56$
   $x = 25.45$ or 25.5 kg

d. lb:kg = lb:kg
   2.2:1 = 21.5:x
   $2.2x = 21.5$
   $x = 9.77$ or 9.8 kg

e. lb:kg = lb:kg
   2.2:1 = 45:x
   $2.2x = 45$
   $x = 20.45$ or 20.5 kg

body surface area

25
---

nomogram

The BSA method, which requires the use of a _____, can be used to determine safe dosage range for infants and children, to calculate dosages specified in mg/M², and to calculate dosages when only the adult dosage is known.

26
---

weight

To determine BSA, you need to know the child's height in inches or centimeters and the _____ in pounds or kilograms.

27

M²

Look at the nomogram printed on the book's back endpapers. To calculate infant and children's BSA, use a ruler to connect the point on the height column (on the left) denoting the child's height, and the point on the weight column (on the right) denoting the child's weight. The point at which the line crosses the BSA column is the body surface area in _____ for that child.

28

0.19

For example, if an infant is 22 inches tall and weighs 5 pounds, the BSA is _____ M².

29

0.5

If a child is 3 feet, 4 inches tall and weighs 20 pounds, the BSA is _____ M².

30
---

surface area in square meters

Again, look at the nomogram. Use the center column of the nomogram, "For Children of Normal Height and Weight," to determine the BSA when the infant or child is not underweight or overweight. The left-hand side of the column represents the weight that corresponds to the right-hand side, indicating _____ _____.

---------------------------------- **31** ----------------------------------

According to the nomogram, a child of normal height weighing 8 pounds has a body surface area of _____ M^2.

0.237

---------------------------------- **32** ----------------------------------

Now You Try It

Determine the BSA using the nomogram on the back inside cover.

a. A child weighs 16 pounds and is 65 centimeters tall. The BSA is _____ M^2.

a. 0.38

b. A child weighs 30 kg and is 50 inches tall. The BSA is _____ M^2.

b. 1.02

c. A child weighs 11 pounds and is 22 inches tall. The BSA is _____ M^2.

c. 0.29

d. A child weighs 20 kg and is 92 centimeters tall. The BSA is _____ M^2.

d. 0.74

Calculating Dosages by Body Surface Area

---------------------------------- **33** ----------------------------------

When the recommended dosage of a drug is given in dosage/M^2 (for example mg/M^2), the specific dosage is multiplied by the BSA to determine safe dosage ranges. For example, the doctor orders "Zovirax 150 mg IV over 1 h," for a child 24 inches tall weighing 40 pounds. The recommended dosage is 250 mg/M^2 IV over 1 h q.8h for five days. The child's BSA, _____ M^2, is multiplied by 250 mg to determine the safe dosage range.

0.6

---------------------------------- **34** ----------------------------------

Using the ratio-and-proportion method to solve the problem, the proportion in units is ____ _____. The numerical proportion is _____. The safe dosage of Zovirox is _____. The prescribed dosage of Zovirox is a _____ dose.

$250{:}1 = x{:}0.6$

$250{:}1 = x{:}0.6$

$x = 250 \times 0.6$
$x = 150 \text{ mg}$

safe

a. 0.8 M²

$1.5:1 = x:0.8$

$x = 1.2$ mg min

$2:1 = x:0.8$

$x = 1.6$ mg max

1.2 mg to 1.6 mg/week

Yes

b. 0.6 M²

$30:1 = x:0.6$

$x = 18$ mg/day

Yes

c. 0.17 M²

$250:1 = x:0.17$

$x = 42.5$ mg/day

No

d. 0.7 M²

$35:1 = x:0.7$

$x = 24.5$ mg min

mg:M² = mg:M²

$45:1 = x:0.7$

$x = 31.5$ mg max

24.5 mg to 31.5 mg/day

Yes

Now You Try It

Using the BSA method, determine if the following doses are safe. Refer to the nomogram to determine BSA.

a. The order reads: Oncovin 1.3 mg IV q. Monday. The child is 52 inches tall and weighs 40 pounds. The recommended dosage is 1.5–2 mg/M²/wk. The BSA is _____. The recommended dosage range is _____. Is the dose therapeutic and safe? _____

b. The order reads: Methotrexate 17.5 mg p.o. today. The child is 92 cm tall and weighs 30 pounds. The recommended dosage is 30 mg/M²/day 2x/week maintenance. The BSA is _____. The maximum safe dosage is _____. Is the dose therapeutic and safe? _____

c. The order reads: 80 mg of a drug IV. The infant is 50 cm tall and weighs 2 kg. The recommended dosage is 250 mg/M² IV. The BSA is _____. The maximum safe dosage is _____. Is the dose therapeutic and safe? _____

d. The order reads: 26 mg of a drug IV. The child is 32 inches tall and weighs 45 pounds. The recommended dosage is 35–45 mg/M²/day in a single dose. The BSA is _____. The recommended dosage range is _____. Is the dose therapeutic and safe? _____

> **REMEMBER**
>
> Read the nomogram carefully. Neither the calibrations nor the increments rise consistently from the bottom of the chart to the top of the chart.

Calculating Pediatric Dosages from Adult Dosages

36

Use the _____ _____ _____ method
to estimate the safe pediatric dosage when only the adult dosage
is known. First, the average adult BSA (1.7 M²) is divided into
the child's BSA. Second, the quotient is multiplied by the adult
dose. Expressed as a formula, the process looks like this:

$$\frac{\text{Child's M}^2}{1.7 \text{ M}^2} \times \text{adult dose} = \text{estimated child's dose}$$

body surface area

37

For example, if the average adult dose of meperidine is 75 mg
IM q.4h p.r.n. and a child's BSA is 0.65 M², the estimated child's
dose is

$$\frac{0.65 \text{M}^2}{1.7 \text{ M}^2} \times 75 \text{ mg} = \text{_____}$$

$\dfrac{0.65 \text{ M}^2}{1.7 \text{ M}^2} \times 75 \text{ mg}$

$= 0.38 \times 75 \text{ mg}$

$= 29 \text{ mg}$

DID YOU NOTICE?

**The calculated child's dose is proportionately smaller than
the average adult dose when the BSA method is used to
estimate a safe dosage.**

38

Now You Try It

Determine the safe child's dose using the BSA formula.

a. The average adult dose is morphine 10 mg q.3h p.r.n. The
child's BSA is 0.75 M². The child's safe dose is _____.

b. The average adult dose is Phenergan 25 mg q.6h IM p.r.n.
nausea. The child's BSA is 0.48 M². The child's safe dose
is _____.

c. The average adult dose is atropine 0.4 mg IM now. The child's
BSA is 0.88 M². The child's safe dose is _____.

a. $\dfrac{0.75 \text{ M}^2}{1.7 \text{ M}^2} \times 10 \text{ mg}$

  $= x$

  $x = 0.44 \times 10 \text{ mg}$

  $x = 4.4 \text{ mg}$

b. $\dfrac{0.48 \text{ M}^2}{1.7 \text{ M}^2} \times 25 \text{ mg}$

  $= x$

  $x = 0.28 \times 25 \text{ mg}$

  $x = 7 \text{ mg}$

c. $\dfrac{0.88 \text{ M}^2}{1.7 \text{ M}^2} \times 0.4 \text{ mg}$

  $= x$

  $x = 0.52 \times 0.4 \text{ mg}$

  $x = 0.2 \text{ mg}$

d. $\dfrac{0.95 \text{ M}^2}{1.7 \text{ M}^2} \times 250 \text{ mg}$

$\quad = x$

$\quad x = 0.56 \times 250 \text{ mg}$

$\quad x = 140 \text{ mg}$

d. The average adult dose is Keflex 250 mg p.o. q.6h. The child's BSA is 0.95 M². The child's safe dose is _____.

Calculating Daily Fluid Needs

39
---

birth / 12

1 / 12

It may be necessary to calculate IV hydration needs for infants (_____ to _____ months) and children (_____ to _____ years) to determine safe limits for fluid intake. The following formulas are accepted for determining the pediatric maintenance IV therapy needs:

1st 10 kg of body weight:	100 mL/kg/24 h
2nd 10 kg of body weight:	50 mL/kg/24 h
Additional weight in kgs:	20 mL/kg/24 h

40

For example, the 24-hour maintenance fluid amount for a 28-kg child would be 1660 mL/24 h. Here's how you determine this amount:

1st 10 kg body weight: 100 mL × 10 kg = 1000 mL

500 mL

2nd 10 kg body weight: 50   mL × 10 kg = _____

Additional weight in kgs: 20   mL × 8   kg = 160 mL

For a total of 1660 mL/24 h.

41

1660 mL ÷ 24 h

$\qquad\qquad = x$

$x = \dfrac{\overset{415}{\cancel{1660} \text{ mL}}}{\underset{6}{\cancel{24} \text{ h}}} = 69 \text{ mL/h}$

69 mL per hour

The IV flow rate (mL/h) needed to deliver 1660 mL/24 h to the child weighing 28 kg is _____. You will set the electronic infusion pump for _____.

REMEMBER

Determine the IV flow rate in mL/h by dividing the total number of hours the infusion is to run into the total amount of solution to be infused.

42

Now You Try It

Determine the following daily fluid needs. Then, determine the hourly IV rate you will set the infusion pump at.

a. The normal daily fluid need of a 7.5-kg infant is _____. You will set the infusion pump at _____.

b. The normal daily fluid need of an 18-kg child is _____. You will set the infusion pump at _____.

c. The normal daily fluid need of a 54-pound child is _____. You will set the infusion pump at _____.

REMEMBER

Convert pounds to kilograms before calculating the daily fluid needs for the pediatric patient.

a. 100 mL × 7.5 kg
    $= x$
    $x = 750$ mL/24 h
    $x = 750$ mL ÷ 24 h
    $x = \dfrac{750 \text{ mL}}{24 \text{ h}}$
    $= \dfrac{31.25 \text{ mL}}{\text{h}}$
    $x = 31$ mL per hour

b. 100 mL × 10
    $= 1000$ mL
    50 mL × 8 kg
    $= 400$ mL
    $x = 1000$ mL +
    400 mL
    $x = 1400$ mL/24 h
    $x = 1400$ mL ÷ 24 h
    $x = 58.33$ mL
    $x = 58$ mL per hour

c. lb:kg = lb:kg
    2.2:1 = 54:x
    $2.2x = 54$
    $x = 24.55$ kg
    45 lbs = 24.6 kg
    100 mL × 10 kg
    $= 1000$ mL
    50 mL × 10 kg
    $= 500$ mL
    20 mL × 4.6 kg
    $= 92$ mL
    $x = 1000 +$
    500 + 92
    $x = 1592$ mL/24 h
    $x = 1592 ÷ 24$ h
    $x = 66.33$/h
    $x = 66$ mL
    per hour

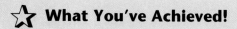
★ You have learned to calculate pediatric dosages using the dosage-per-kilogram-of-body-weight and the body-surface-area methods.

★ You can calculate body surface areas.

★ You know how to verify safe dosages by comparing recommended dosages to prescribed dosages.

Terrific! What you've learned in this chapter will help you determine pediatric drug dosages and verify safe dosages for the pediatric patient. Before moving forward, take the review test to demonstrate your mastery of drug dosage considerations for the pediatric patient. If you get more than one wrong in any section, consider studying that portion of the chapter again.

Review Test

─── A ───

Complete the following statements or answer the following questions.

1. Physiologic maturity has a great impact on _____, _____, _____, and _____ of medications.

2. The two most accurate ways to calculate pediatric dosage ranges are the _____ _____ _____ _____ _____ _____ and _____ _____ _____ methods.

3. The age range for an infant is _____, and for a child is _____.

4. A _____ is used to determine body surface area which is designated by the abbreviation _____.

Change the following pounds to kilograms. Round your answer to the nearest tenth.

5. 18 pounds = _____ kilograms   6. 64 pounds = _____ kilograms

Answer the following questions comparing prescribed dosage to recommended dosage using the dosage-per-kilogram-of-body-weight method.

7. The order reads: Ceclor 300 mg p.o. q.12h. The child weighs 22 kg and the recommended dosage of Ceclor is 20–40 mg/kg/day, q.12h doses. The dosage range is _____. What is the divided dosage range? _____ Is the dose safe? _____

8. The order reads: penicillin V 500,000 U p.o. q.6h. The child weighs 20 kg and the recommended dosage for penicillin V is 25,000–90,000 U/kg/day in 4 divided doses. The dosage range is _____. What is the divided dosage range? _____ Is the dose safe? _____

9. The order reads: dicloxacillin 300 mg p.o. q.6h. The child weighs 38.5 pounds and the recommended dosage is dicloxacillin, 12.5–25 mg/kg q.6h. The child's weight in kg is _____. What is the dosage range? _____. What is the divided dosage range? _____ Is the dose safe? _____

10. The order reads: gentamicin 40 mg IV q.8h. The child weighs 44 pounds and the recommended dosage is gentamicin, 2–2.5 mg/kg q.8h. The child's weight in kg is _____. What is the divided dosage range? _____ Is the dose safe? _____

Determine if the following ordered dosages are safe, using the BSA method.

11. The order reads: Cytosar 150 mg IV. The child's BSA is 0.97 M^2 and the recommended dosage is Cytosar, 100 mg/M^2/day × 5–10 days. The safe dose is _____. Is the ordered dose safe? _____

12. The order reads: Cytoxan 90 mg IV. The child's BSA is 0.66 M^2 and the recommended dosage is 60–250 mg/M^2/day for 6–7 days. The safe dose is _____. Is the ordered dose safe? _____

Calculate the following daily fluid needs.

13. The daily fluid requirement for a 17-kg child is _____. The hourly IV rate is _____.

14. The 24-hour maintenance fluid requirement for a 12-lb child is _____. The hourly IV rate is _____.

— F —

Determine the safe dose for a child, using the BSA method and the known adult average dose.

15. If the average adult dose is Dilantin 100 mg p.o. t.i.d., and the child's BSA is 0.9 M², the child's maximum dose is _____.

16. If the average adult dose is nafcillin 500 mg p.o. q.6h, and the child's BSA is 0.83 M², the child's maximum dose is _____.

17. If the average adult dose is Mysoline 250 mg p.o. q.i.d., and the child's BSA is 0.54 M², the child's maximum dose is _____.

18. If the average adult dose is Clindamycin 300 mg IV q.6h, and the child's BSA is 0.32 M², the child's maximum dose is _____.

Answers for Review Test

1. absorption, distribution, metabolism, and excretion

2. dosage-per-kilogram-of-body-weight and body-surface-area

3. birth to 12 months, 1 to 12 years   4. nomogram, M²

5. lb:kg = lb:kg

$$2.2:1 = 18:x$$

$$\frac{2.2x}{2.2} = \frac{18}{2.2}$$

$$x = 8.2 \text{ kg}$$

6. lb:kg = lb:kg

$$2.2:1 = 64:x$$

$$\frac{2.2x}{2.2} = \frac{64}{2.2}$$

$$x = 29.1 \text{ kg}$$

7. mg:kg = mg:kg   mg:kg = mg:kg

   $20:1 = x:22$ $40:1 = x:22$

   $x = 440$ mg min $x = 880$ mg max

   Dosage range = 440 mg to 880 mg

   $440 \div 2 = 220$ mg, $880 \div 2 = 440$ mg

   Divided dosage range = 220 mg to 440 mg

   Yes

---

8.   U:kg = U:kg   U:kg = U:kg

   $25,000:1 = x:20$ $90,000:1 = 20:x$

   $x = 500,000$ U min $x = 1,800,000$ U max

   Dosage range = 500,000 U to 1,800,000 U

   Divided minimum is 500,000 U $\div$ 4 = 125,000 U

   Divided maximum is 1,800,000 U $\div$ 4 = 450,000 U

   Divided dosage range = 125,000 U to 450,000 U

   No

---

9. lb:kg = lb:kg

   $2.2:1 = 38.5:x$

   $\dfrac{\cancel{2.2}x}{\cancel{2.2}} = \dfrac{38.5}{2.2}$

   $x = 17.5$ kg

   mg:kg = mg:kg   mg:kg = mg:kg

   $12.5:1 = x:17.5$ $25:1 = x:17.5$

   $x = 218.8$ mg min $x = 437.5$ mg max

   Divided dosage range = 218.8 mg to 437.5 mg

   Yes

---

10. lb:kg = lb:kg

$$2.2{:}1 = 44{:}x$$

$$\frac{2.2x}{2.2} = \frac{44}{2.2}$$

$$x = 20 \text{ kg}$$

mg:kg = mg:kg   mg:kg = mg:kg

$$2{:}1 = x{:}20 \qquad\qquad 2.5{:}1 = x{:}20$$

$$x = 40 \text{ mg min} \qquad x = 50 \text{ mg max}$$

    Divided dosage range = 40 mg to 50 mg

    Yes

---

11. $mg{:}M^2 = mg{:}M^2$

$$100{:}1 = x{:}0.97$$

$$x = 97 \text{ mg}$$

    Recommended dose is 97 mg

    No

12. $mg{:}M^2 = mg{:}M^2 \qquad mg{:}M^2 = mg{:}M^2$

$$60{:}1 = x{:}0.66 \qquad 250{:}1 = x{:}0.66$$

$$x = 39.6 \text{ mg min} \qquad x = 165 \text{ mg max}$$

    Dosage range is 39.6 mg to 165 mg

    Yes

---

13. $x = 100 \text{ mL} \times 10 \text{ kg} = 1000 \text{ mL}$

    $x = 50 \text{ mL} \times 7 \text{ kg} = 350 \text{ mL}$

    $x = 1000 \text{ mL} + 350 \text{ mL} = 1350 \text{ mL/24 h}$

    $x = 1350 \text{ mL} \div 24 \text{ h} = 56.25 \text{ mL/h} = 56 \text{ mL per hour}$

---

14. lb:kg = lb:kg

$$2.2{:}1 = 12{:}x$$

$$2.2x = 12$$

$$x = 5.45 \text{ kg}$$

$$x = 100 \text{ mL} \times 5.45 \text{ kg} = 545 \text{ mL/24 h}$$

$$x = 545 \text{ mL} \div 24 \text{ h} = 22.71 \text{ mL/h} = 23 \text{ mL per hour}$$

---

15. $\dfrac{0.9 \text{ M}^2}{1.7 \text{ M}^2} \times 100 \text{ mg} = x$

    $0.53 \times 100 \text{ mg} = 53 \text{ mg child's dose}$

---

16. $\dfrac{0.83 \text{ M}^2}{1.7 \text{ M}^2} \times 500 \text{ mg} = x$

    $0.49 \times 500 \text{ mg} = 245 \text{ mg child's dose}$

---

17. $\dfrac{0.54 \text{ M}^2}{1.7 \text{ M}^2} \times 250 \text{ mg} = x$

    $0.32 \times 250 \text{ mg} = 80 \text{ mg child's dose}$

---

18. $\dfrac{0.32 \text{ M}^2}{1.7 \text{ M}^2} \times 300 \text{ mg} = x$

    $0.19 \times 300 \text{ mg} = 57 \text{ mg child's dose}$

V

COMPREHENSIVE EXAM

⭐ CONGRATULATIONS! YOU HAVE COMPLETED *QuickCalc* and now should have the skills necessary to calculate drug dosages with confidence and accuracy.

Take the comprehensive examination that begins on the next page to evaluate your mastery of dosage calculation skills. The exam is divided into seven sections for a total of 85 problems. You should complete the exam in 2.5 hours with at least a 90% score, or 75 correct problems. If you get more than two answers wrong in any section, turn to the chapter in the book and review those sections that correspond to the content area of the incorrect responses.

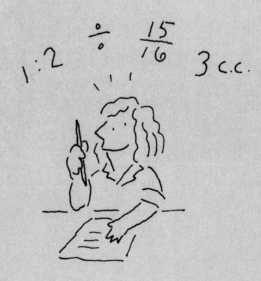

Systems of Measurement

Calculate the following equivalents. (Complete in 15 minutes.)

1. 336 mg   = _____ g

2. 0.025 mg = _____ mcg

3. 75 mL   = _____ L

4. A premature infant weighs 9.095 kg. How many grams is this?   _____

5. A physician orders atropine 400 mcg. How many milligrams is this?   _____

6. A patient drinks 1.350 L. How many milliliters is this?   _____

7. A physician orders Motrin 0.8 g. How many milligrams is this?   _____

8. A physician orders 650 mg of acetaminophen. How many grams is this?   _____

9. F℥ $1\frac{2}{3}$ = _____ ℳ

10. F℥ xxiv = _____ f℥

11. ℳ 360   = _____ f℥

12. A patient receives f℥$\frac{3}{4}$ castor oil. How many fluidrams is this?   _____

13. A physician orders f℥ iss. How many minims is this?   _____

14. 5 tsp = _____ T

15. 15 gtt = _____ t

16. 3 T   = _____ f℥

Conversion Between Systems of Measurement

Calculate the following equivalents. (Complete in 15 minutes.)

17. ℥ XII   = _____ mL

18. gr vss   = _____ mg

19. 2.4 mL = _____ ℥

20. 8 gtt   = _____ ℥

21. 3.5 T   = _____ mL

22. 145 lb = _____ kg

23. 65 kg   = _____ lb

24. A physician orders Scopolamine 1 mg. How many grains is this?   _____

25. A physician orders NPH 75 U. How many milligrams is this?   _____

26. A patient drinks $5\frac{2}{3}$ fluidounces of juice. How many milliliters is this?   _____

27. A patient weights 198 pounds. How many kilograms is this?   _____

28. A patient weighs 75 kg. How many pounds is this?   _____

29. A patient is to receive 4 tsp of Metamucil. How many milliliters is this?   _____

30. The physician orders "push fluids to 3000 mL/day." How many 8-ounce glasses is this?

_____

Oral Medications

Calculate the following oral medication dosages. Use the medication labels provided or the available dosage. (Complete in 35 minutes.)

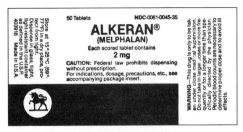

FIGURE E.1

31. Trade name: _____
Generic name: _____
Dosage form: _____
Dosage strength: _____
The order reads: Alkeran 6 mg p.o. q.d.
Amount administered: _____

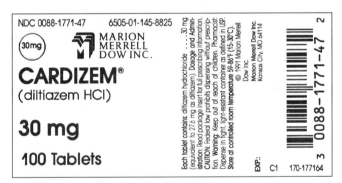

FIGURE E.2

32. Trade name: _____
Generic name: _____
Dosage form: _____
Dosage strength: _____
The order reads: Cardizem 120 mg p.o. b.i.d.
Amount administered: _____

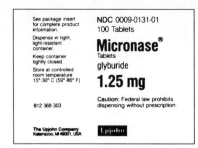

FIGURE E.3

33. Trade name: _____
    Generic name: _____
    Dosage form: _____
    Dosage strength: _____
    The order reads: Micronase 3.75 mg q.d.
    Amount administered: _____

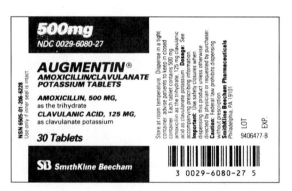

FIGURE E.4

34. Trade name: _____
    Generic name: _____
    Dosage form: _____
    Dosage strength: _____
    The order reads: Augmentin 0.5 g p.o. q.8h
    Amount administered: _____

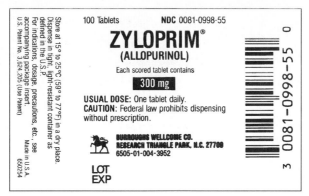

FIGURE E.5

35. The order reads: Zyloprim 450 mg p.o. q.d.
Amount administered: _____

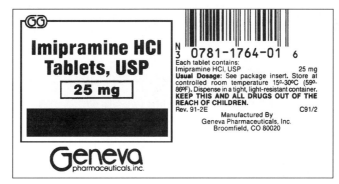

FIGURE E.6

36. The order reads: imipramine 75 mg p.o. h.s.
Amount administered: _____

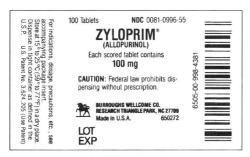

FIGURE E.7

37. The order reads: allopurinol 0.3 g p.o. q.d.
Amount administered: _____

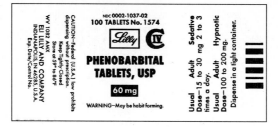

FIGURE E.8

38. The order reads: phenobarbitol gr II p.o. q.d.
Amount administered: _____

39. The order reads: penicillin G potassium 500,000 U p.o. q.8h
Drug available: penicillin G potassium 200,000 U/5 mL
Amount administered: _____

40. The order reads: Mycostatin 400,000 U p.o. q.i.d.
Drug available: Mycostatin 500,000 U/5 mL
Amount administered: _____

41. The order reads: levothyroxine 0.225 mg p.o. q.d.
Drug available: levothyroxine 75 mcg/tab
Amount administered: _____

42. The order reads: Tylenol gr viiss p.o. q.4h p.r.n.
Drug available: Tylenol 500 mg/5 mL
Amount administered: _____

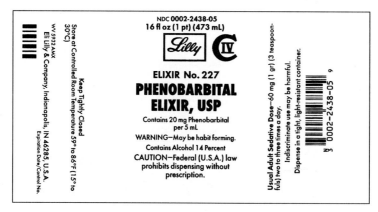

FIGURE E.9

43. The order reads: phenobarbitol gr $\frac{3}{4}$ p.o. t.i.d.
Amount administered: _____

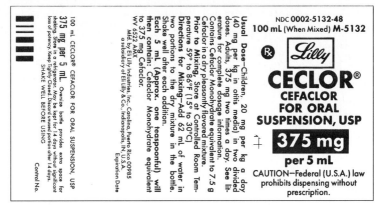

FIGURE E.10

44. The order reads: Ceclor 300 mg p.o. q.8h
Reconstitute with: _____
Dosage strength: _____
Amount administered: _____

45. The order reads: Augmentin 0.375 g p.o.
Reconstitute with 75 mL water.
Dosage strength is 250 mg/5 mL
Amount administered: _____

Parenteral Medications

Calculate the following dosages using the medication labels or available dosages. (Complete in 30 minutes.)

46. The order reads: Demerol 45 mg IM q.4h p.r.n.
Drug available: Demerol 50 mg/mL
Amount administered: _____

47. The order reads: Calcimar 125 U IM
Drug available: Calcimar 100 U/mL
Amount administered: _____

48. The order reads: cortisone 75 mg IM
Drug available: cortisone 50 mg/mL
Amount administered: _____

49. The order reads: Inapsine 3.5 mg IM @ 8 a.m.
    Drug available: Inapsine 2.5 mg/mL
    Amount administered: _____

50. The order reads: Buprenex 0.5 mg q.6h p.r.n. pain
    Drug available: Buprenex 300 mcg/mL
    Amount administered: _____

51. The order reads: Rubramin 300 mcg IM q.month
    Drug available: Rubramin 0.120 mg/mL
    Amount administered: _____

52. The order reads: phenobarbitol 90 mg IM q.8h
    Drug available: phenobarbitol gr I/mL
    Amount administered: _____

53. The order reads: Toradol 45 mg IM q.6h
    Drug available: Toradol 2 mL cartridge (30 mg/mL)
    Amount administered: _____

54. The order reads: morphine 10 mg IM q.3h p.r.n.
    Drug available: morphine gr $\frac{1}{4}$/mL
    Amount administered: _____

55. The order reads: Staphcillin 1.25 g IM q.6h
    Drug available: Staphcillin 500 mg/mL
    Amount administered: _____

56. The order reads: clindamycin 225 mg IM q.6h
    Drug available: clindamycin 150 mg/mL
    Amount administered: _____

57. The order reads: Nembutol 80 mg IM h.s.
    Drug available: Nembutol 50 mg/mL
    Amount administered: _____

58. The order reads: penicillin G 900,000 U IM
    Drug available: penicillin G 600,000 U/mL
    Amount administered: _____

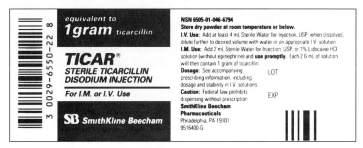

FIGURE E.11

59. The order reads: Ticar 600 mg q.4h IM
Reconstitute with: _____
Dosage strength: _____
Amount administered: _____

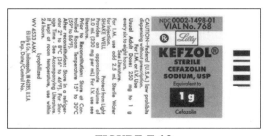

FIGURE E.12

60. The order reads: Kefzol 0.66 g IM q.8h
Reconstitute with: _____
Dosage strength: _____
Amount administered: _____

Syringe Interpretation

Draw an arrow on each syringe to indicate the measured amount of medication to administer. (Complete in 10 minutes.)

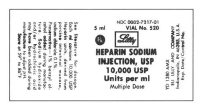

FIGURE E.13

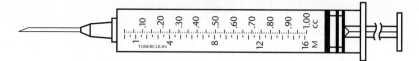

FIGURE E.14

61. The order reads: heparin 6500 U SQ
Amount administered: _____

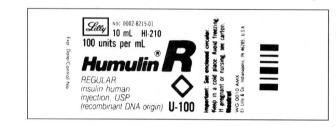

FIGURE E.15

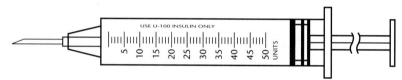

FIGURE E.16

62. The order reads: Humulin R 28 U SQ q.a.m.
Amount administered: _____

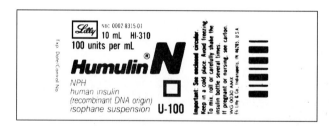

FIGURE E.17

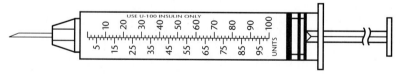

FIGURE E.18

63. The order reads: Humulin N 57 U SQ
Amount administered: _____

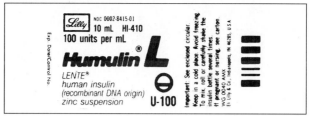

FIGURE E.19

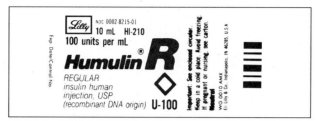

FIGURE E.20

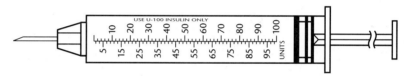

FIGURE E.21

64. The order reads: Humulin L 40 U & Humulin R 12 U this a.m.
Amount administered: _____

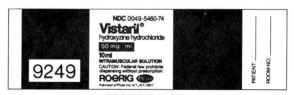

FIGURE E.22

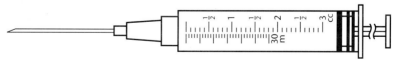

FIGURE E.23

65. The order reads: Vistaril 65 mg IM q.4h p.r.n. nausea
Amount administered: _____

Intravenous Medications

Calculate the following rates. (Complete in 20 minutes.)

66. The order reads: D5W 250 mL IV over 6 h
    Drop factor: 60 gtt/mL
    Flow rate, gtt/min: _____

67. The order reads: D5W 1000 mL q.12h IV
    Drop factor: 20 gtt/mL
    Flow rate, gtt/min: _____

68. The order reads: D5 0.45 NS 3000 mL/24 h
    Drop factor: 15 gtt/mL
    Flow rate, gtt/min: _____

69. The order reads: ticarcillin 2 g q.8h IVPB, mix in 100 mL D5W, infuse over 45 minutes
    Drop factor: 15 gtt/mL
    Flow rate, gtt/min: _____

70. The order reads: Ticar 3 g q.6h IVPB, mix in 75 mL D5W, infuse over 30 minutes
    Drop factor: 10 gtt/mL
    Flow rate, gtt/min: _____

71. The order reads: D5 Ringer's lactate 1000 mL IV q.8h was started @ 8 a.m.
    Drop factor: 15 gtt/mL
    Flow rate, gtt/min: _____
    At 1 p.m. 435 mL remain. The flow rate in gtt/min must be increased to _____
    to complete the IV on time.

72. The order reads: D5W 1000 mL IV over 10 hours
    Drop factor: 20 gtt/mL
    Flow rate, gtt/min: _____
    After 6 hours 325 mL remain. The new flow rate, gtt/min, to complete IV on time
    is _____.

73. The order reads: heparin 25,000 U in 1000 mL D5W IV to infuse @ 2000 U/h
    Flow rate, mL/h: _____
    Electronic IV infusion pump is set at: _____

74. The order reads: D5W 500 mL IV with 20,000 U heparin to infuse @ 1200 U/h
    Flow rate, mL/h: _____

75. The order reads: NSS 500 mL to run @ 45 mL/h
    How many hours will the infusion last?   _____

Pediatric Dosages

Calculate the following problems. (Complete in 25 minutes.)

76. The order reads: chlorothiazide 500 mg p.o. b.i.d. (twice/day)
    Child's weight: 55 kg
    Recommended dose: p.o., 20 mg/kg/day in divided doses
    Dosage/day: _____
    Divided dose: _____
    Is dose safe?   _____

77. The order reads: Pyridium 100 mg p.o. t.i.d.
    Child's weight: 30 kg
    Recommended dose: p.o., 12 mg/kg/day, divided doses
    Dosage/day: _____
    Divided dose: _____
    Is dose safe?   _____

78. The order reads: clindamycin 300 mg p.o. q.6h
    Child's weight: 35 kg
    Recommended dose: p.o., 8–25 mg/kg/day, q.6h
    Dosage range: _____
    Divided dosage range: _____
    Is dose safe?   _____

79. The order reads: Decadron 1.5 mg p.o. q.i.d. (4x day)
    Child's weight: 30 kg
    Recommended dose: 0.2 mg/kg/day, q.6h
    Dosage/day: _____
    Divided dose: _____
    Is dose safe?   _____

80. The order reads: E.E.S. 250 mg p.o. q.i.d.
    Child's weight: 25 kg
    Recommended dose: 30–50 mg/kg/day, q.6h
    Dosage range: _____
    Divided dosage range: _____
    Is dose safe?   _____

81. The order reads: flucytosine 0.5 g p.o. q.6h
BSA: 0.74 M^2
Recommended dose: p.o., 1.5–4.5g/M^2/day in 4 divided doses
Dosage range: _____
Divided dosage range: _____
Is dose safe? _____

82. The order reads: lomustine 125 mg IV q.8h
BSA: 0.56 M^2
Recommended dose: IV, 250 mg/M^2/q.8h for 1 week
Dosage/day: _____
Is dose safe? _____

83. Average adult dose: ferrous sulfate 325 mg p.o. t.i.d.
Child's BSA: 1.4 M^2
Child's maximum dose: _____

84. Average adult dose: Phenergan 25 mg IM q.6h p.r.n. nausea
Child's BSA: 0.38 M^2
Child's maximum dose: _____

85. Average adult dose: Benadryl 50 mg p.o. q.4–6h p.r.n.
Child's BSA: 0.75 M^2
Child's maximum dose: _____

Answers for Comprehensive Examination

Systems of Measurement

Review found in Chapter 5.

1. mg:g = mg:g

    $1000:1 = 336:x$

    $1000x = 336$

    $x = 0.336$ g

2. mg:mcg = mg:mcg

    $1:1000 = 0.025:x$

    $x = 25$ mcg

3. mL:L = mL:L

    $1000:1 = 75:x$

    $1000x = 75$

    $x = 0.075$ L

4. g:kg = g:kg

    $1000:1 = x:9.095$

    $x = 9095$ g

5. mg:mcg = mg:mcg

    $1:1000 = x:400$

    $1000x = 400$

    $x = 0.4$ mg

6. mL:L = mL:L

    $1000:1 = x:1.350$

    $x = 1350$ mL

7.
$$mg:g = mg:g$$
$$1000:1 = x:0.8$$
$$x = 800 \text{ mg}$$

8.
$$mg:g = mg:g$$
$$1000:1 = 650:x$$
$$1000x = 650$$
$$x = 0.65 \text{ g}$$

Review found in Chapter 6.

9.
$$fℨ:ℳ = fℨ:ℳ$$
$$1:480 = 1\tfrac{2}{3}:x$$
$$x = 480 \times \tfrac{5}{3} = 800 \text{ ℳ}$$

10.
$$fʒ:fℨ = fʒ:fℨ$$
$$8:1 = 24:x$$
$$8x = 24$$
$$x = fℨ \text{ iii}$$

11.
$$ℳ:fʒ = ℳ:fʒ$$
$$480:1 = 360:x$$
$$480x = 360$$
$$x = fʒ \tfrac{3}{4}$$

12.
$$fʒ:fℨ = fʒ:fℨ$$
$$1:8 = \tfrac{3}{4}:x$$
$$x = fʒ \text{ vi}$$

13.
$$ℳ:fʒ = ℳ:fʒ$$
$$60:1 = x:1.5$$
$$x = ℳ \text{ 90}$$

Review found in Chapter 7.

14.
$$tsp:T = tsp:T$$
$$3:1 = 5:x$$
$$3x = 5$$
$$x = 1\tfrac{2}{3} \text{ T}$$

15.
$$gtt:t = gtt:t$$
$$60:1 = 15:x$$
$$60x = 15$$
$$x = \tfrac{1}{4} \text{ t}$$

16.
$$T:fʒ = T:fʒ$$
$$2:1 = 3:x$$
$$2x = 3$$
$$x = fʒ \text{ iss}$$

Conversion Between Systems

Review found in Chapter 8.

17.
$$mL:ℳ = mL:ℳ$$
$$1:16 = x:12$$
$$16x = 12$$
$$x = 0.75 \text{ mL}$$

18.
$$mg:gr = mg:gr$$
$$60:1 = x:5.5$$
$$x = 330 \text{ mg}$$

19.
$$mL:ℳ = mL:ℳ$$
$$1:15 = 2.4:x$$
$$x = 36 \text{ ℳ}$$

20. 1 gtt = ♏ I
8 gtt = ♏ VIII

21. mL:T = mL:T

$15:1 = x:3.5$

$x = 52.5$ cc

22. kg:lb = kg:lb

$1:2.2 = x:145$

$2.2x = 145$

$x = 65.9$ kg

---

23. kg:lb = kg:lb

$1:2.2 = 65:x$

$x = 143$ lb

24. mg:gr = mg:gr

$60:1 = 1:x$

$60x = 1$

$x = \text{gr } \dfrac{1}{60}$

25. Units do not equate to milligrams.

---

26. mL:f℥ = mL:f℥

$30:1 = x:5\dfrac{2}{3}$

$x = 30 \times \dfrac{17}{3}$

$x = 170$ mL

27. kg:lb = kg:lb

$1:2.2 = x:198$

$2.2x = 198$

$x = 90$ kg

28. kg:lb = kg:lb

$1:2.2 = 75:x$

$x = 165$ lb

---

29. mL:t = mL:t

$5:1 = x:4$

$x = 20$ mL

30. f℥:mL = f℥:mL

$1:30 = x:3000$

$30x = 3000$

$x = 100$ f℥

f℥ 100 ÷ 8 = 12.5 glasses

Oral Medications

Review found in Chapters 9 and 10.

31. Alkeran, melphalan, scored tablet, 2 mg/tablet

mg:tab = mg:tab

$2:1 = 6:x$

$2x = 6$

$x = 3$ tablets

32. Cardizem, diltiazem, tablet, 30 mg/tablet

mg:tab = mg:tab

$30:1 = 120:x$

$30x = 120$

$x = 4$ tablets

---

33. Micronase, glyburide, tablet, 1.25 mg/tablet

mg:tab = mg:tab

$1.25{:}1 = 3.75{:}x$

$1.25x = 3.75$

$x = 3$ tablets

34. Augmentin, amoxicillin, tablet, 500 mg/tablet

mg:g = mg:g

$1000{:}1 = x{:}0.5$

$x = 500$ mg

mg:tab = mg:tab

$500{:}1 = 500{:}x$

$500x = 500$

$x = 1$ tablet

---

35. mg:tab = mg:tab

$300{:}1 = 450{:}x$

$300x = 450$

$x = 1.5$ scored tablet

36. mg:tab = mg:tab

$25{:}1 = 75{:}x$

$25x = 75$

$x = 3$ tablets

37. mg:g = mg:g

$1000{:}1 = x = 0.3$

$x = 300$ mg

mg:tab = mg:tab

$100{:}1 = 300{:}x$

$100x = 300$

$x = 3$ tablets

---

38. mg:gr = mg:gr

$60{:}1 = x{:}2$

$x = 120$ mg

mg:tab = mg:tab

$60{:}1 = 120{:}x$

$60x = 120$

$x = 2$ tablets

39. U:mL = U:mL

$200{,}000{:}5 = 500{,}000{:}x$

$200{,}000x = 2{,}500{,}000$

$x = 12.5$ mL

40. U:mL = U:mL

$500{,}000{:}5 = 400{,}000{:}x$

$500{,}000x = 2{,}000{,}000$

$x = 4$ mL

---

41. mcg:mg = mcg:mg

$1000:1 = x{:}0.225$

$x = 225$ mcg

mcg:tab = mcg:tab

$75:1 = 225{:}x$

$75x = 225$

$x = 3$ tablets

42. mg:gr = mg:gr

$60:1 = x{:}7.5$

$x = 450$ mg

mg:mL = mg:mL

$500:5 = 450{:}x$

$500x = 2250$

$x = 4.5$ mL

43. mg:gr = mg:gr

$60:1 = x{:}\dfrac{3}{4}$

$x = 45$ mg

mg:mL = mg:mL

$20:5 = 45{:}x$

$20x = 225$

$x = 11.25$ mL

44. 62 mL water

375 mg/5 mL

mg:mL = mg:mL

$375:5 = 300{:}x$

$375x = 1500$

$x = 4$ mL

Parenteral Medications

Review found in Chapter 11.

45. mg:g = mg:g

$1000:1 = x{:}0.375$

$x = 375$ mg

mg:mL = mg:mL

$250:5 = 375{:}x$

$250x = 1875$

$x = 7.5$ mL

46. mg:mL = mg:mL

$50:1 = 45{:}x$

$50x = 45$

$x = 0.9$ mL

47. U:mL = U:mL

$100:1 = 125{:}x$

$100x = 125$

$x = 1.25$ mL

48. mg:mL = mg:mL

$50:1 = 75{:}x$

$50x = 75$

$x = 1.5$ mL

49. mg:mL = mg:mL

$2.5:1 = 3.5{:}x$

$2.5x = 3.5$

$x = 1.4$ mL

50. mcg:mg = mcg:mg

$1000:1 = x:0.5$

$x = 500$ mcg

mcg:mL = mcg:mL

$300:1 = 500:x$

$300x = 500$

$x = 1.67$ mL

51. mcg:mg = mcg:mg

$1000:1 = x:0.120$

$x = 120$ mcg

mcg:mL = mcg:mL

$120:1 = 300:x$

$120x = 300$

$x = 2.5$ mL

52. mg:mL = mg:mL

$60:1 = 90:x$

$60x = 90$

$x = 1.5$ mL

53. mg:mL = mg:mL

$30:1 = 45:x$

$30x = 45$

$x = 1.5$ mL

54. mg:gr = mg:gr

$60:1 = x:0.25$

$x = 15$ mg

mg:mL = mg:mL

$15:1 = 10:x$

$15x = 10$

$x = 0.67$ mL

55. mg:g = mg:g

$1000:1 = x:1.25$

$x = 1250$ mg

mg:mL = mg:mL

$500:1 = 1250:x$

$500x = 1250$

$x = 2.5$ mL

56. mg:mL = mg:mL

$150:1 = 225:x$

$150x = 225$

$x = 1.5$ mL

57. mg:mL = mg:mL

$50:1 = 80:x$

$x = 1.6$ mL

58. U:mL = U:mL

$600,000:1 = 900,000:x$

$600,000x = 900,000$

$x = 1.5$ mL

59. 2 mL sterile water

1 g/2.6 mL

$1g = 1000$ mg

mg:mL = mg:mL

$1000:2.6 = 600:x$

$1000x = 1560$

$x = 1.56$ mL

60. 2.5 mL sterile water

330 mg/mL

mg:g = mg:g

$1000:1 = x:0.66$

$x = 660$ mg

mg:mL = mg:mL

$330:1 = 660:x$

$330x = 660$

$x = 2$ mL

Syringe Interpretation

Review found in Chapter 11.

61.   U:cc = U:cc

10,000:1 = 6500:x

10,000x = 6500

x = 0.65 cc

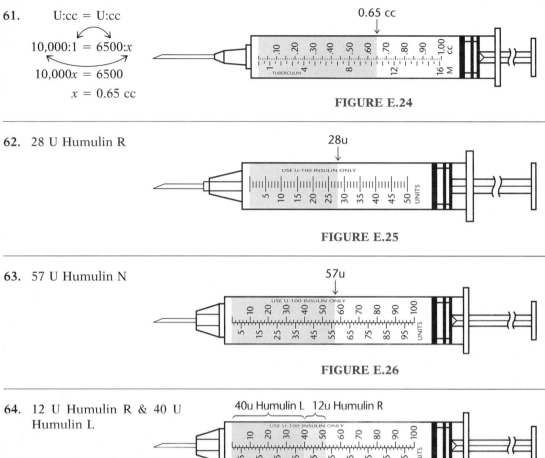

0.65 cc

FIGURE E.24

62. 28 U Humulin R

28u

FIGURE E.25

63. 57 U Humulin N

57u

FIGURE E.26

64. 12 U Humulin R & 40 U Humulin L

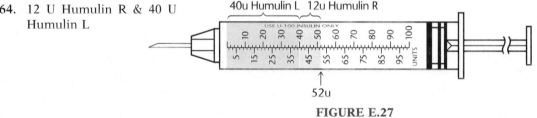

40u Humulin L   12u Humulin R

52u

FIGURE E.27

65. mg:mL = mg:mL

50:1 = 65:x

50x = 65

x = 1.3 mL

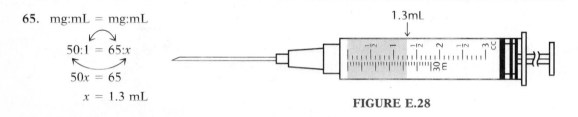

1.3mL

FIGURE E.28

Intravenous Medications

Review in Chapter 13.

66. $\dfrac{250 \text{ mL}}{6 \text{ h}} \times \dfrac{1 \text{ h}}{60 \text{ min}} \times \dfrac{60 \text{ gtt}}{1 \text{ mL}} = 41.7$ gtt/min or 42 gtt/min

---

67. $\dfrac{\overset{250}{\cancel{1000}} \text{ mL}}{\underset{3}{\cancel{12}} \text{ h}} \times \dfrac{1 \text{ h}}{\underset{3}{\cancel{60}} \text{ min}} \times \dfrac{\overset{1}{\cancel{20}} \text{ gtt}}{1 \text{ mL}} = \dfrac{250 \text{ gtt}}{9 \text{ min}} = 27.8$ gtt/min or 28 gtt/min

---

68. $\dfrac{\overset{\overset{250}{\cancel{1000}}}{\cancel{3000}} \text{ mL}}{\underset{8}{\cancel{24}} \text{ h}} \times \dfrac{1 \text{ h}}{\underset{\underset{1}{\cancel{4}}}{\cancel{60}} \text{ min}} \times \dfrac{\overset{1}{\cancel{15}} \text{ gtt}}{1 \text{ mL}} = \dfrac{250 \text{ gtt}}{8 \text{ min}} = 31.3$ gtt/min or 31 gtt/min

---

69. $\dfrac{100 \text{ mL}}{\underset{3}{\cancel{45}} \text{ min}} \times \dfrac{\overset{1}{\cancel{15}} \text{ gtt}}{1 \text{ mL}} = 33$ gtt/min

70. $\dfrac{75 \text{ mL}}{\underset{3}{\cancel{30}} \text{ min}} \times \dfrac{\overset{1}{\cancel{10}} \text{ gtt}}{1 \text{ mL}} = 25$ gtt/min

---

71. $\dfrac{\overset{250}{\cancel{1000}} \text{ mL}}{8 \text{ h}} \times \dfrac{1 \text{ h}}{\underset{\underset{1}{\cancel{4}}}{\cancel{60}} \text{ min}} \times \dfrac{\overset{1}{\cancel{15}} \text{ gtt}}{1 \text{ mL}} = 31$ gtt/min

$\dfrac{\overset{145}{\cancel{435}} \text{ mL}}{\underset{1}{\cancel{3}} \text{ h}} \times \dfrac{1 \text{ h}}{\underset{4}{\cancel{60}} \text{ min}} \times \dfrac{\overset{1}{\cancel{15}} \text{ gtt}}{1 \text{ mL}} = 36$ gtt/mL

---

72. $\dfrac{\overset{100}{\cancel{1000}} \text{ mL}}{\underset{1}{\cancel{10}} \text{ h}} \times \dfrac{1 \text{ h}}{\underset{3}{\cancel{60}} \text{ min}} \times \dfrac{\overset{1}{\cancel{20}} \text{ gtt}}{1 \text{ mL}} = 33$ gtt/min

$\dfrac{325 \text{ mL}}{4 \text{ h}} \times \dfrac{1 \text{ h}}{\underset{3}{\cancel{60}} \text{ min}} \times \dfrac{\overset{1}{\cancel{20}} \text{ gtt}}{1 \text{ mL}} = \dfrac{325 \text{ gtt}}{12 \text{ min}} = 27$ gtt/min

---

73.

$$\frac{2000 \text{ U}}{1 \text{ h}} \times \frac{\overset{40}{\cancel{1000}} \text{ mL}}{\underset{1}{\cancel{25000}} \text{ U}} = 80 \text{ mL/h}$$

74.

$$\frac{6}{\cancel{1200} \cancel{U}} \times \frac{500 \text{ mL}}{\underset{1}{\cancel{20000} \cancel{U}}} = 30 \text{ mL/h}$$

75.

$$\frac{\overset{100}{\cancel{500} \cancel{mL}}}{1} \times \frac{1 \text{ h}}{\underset{9}{\cancel{45} \cancel{mL}}} = 11.1 \text{ hours}$$

Pediatric Dosages

Review found in Chapter 14.

---

76. mg:kg = mg:kg
  20:1 = x:55
    x = 1100 mg
  550 mg/dose, Yes

---

77. mg:kg = mg:kg
  12:1 = x:30
    x = 360 mg
  120 mg/dose, Yes

---

78. mg:kg = mg:kg
    8:1 = x:35
      x = 280 mg (min)

  mg:kg = mg:kg
    25:1 = x:35
      x = 875 mg (max)
  280–875 mg
  280 mg ÷ 4 = 70 mg (min)
  875 mg ÷ 4 = 218.8 mg (max), 70–218.8 mg
  No, too high, hold and consult with physician

---

79. mg:kg = mg:kg
    0.2:1 = x:30
      x = 6 mg
  6 mg ÷ 4 = 1.5 mg
  Yes

---

80. mg:kg = mg:kg
    30:1 = x:25
        x = 750 mg (min)

    mg:kg = mg:kg
    50:1 = x:25
        x = 1250 mg (max)
    750–1250 mg
    750 mg ÷ 4 = 187.5 mg (min)
    1250 mg ÷ 4 = 312.5 mg (max)
    187.5–312.5 mg
    Yes

---

81. g:M^2 = g:M^2
    1.5:1 = x:0.74
        x = 1.1 g (min)

    g:M^2 = g:M^2
    4.5:1 = x:0.74
        x = 3.3 g (max)
    1.1–3.3 g
    1.1 g ÷ 4 = 0.275 g (min)
    3.3 g ÷ 4 = 0.833 g (max)   0.275–0.833 g
    Yes

---

82. mg:M^2 = mg:M^2
    250:1 = x:0.56
        x = 140 mg

    Yes

---

83. $\dfrac{1.4 \ \cancel{M^2}}{1.7 \ \cancel{M^2}} \times 325 \text{ mg} = 0.82 \times 325 \text{ mg} = 267 \text{ mg}$

---

84. $\dfrac{0.38 \ \cancel{M^2}}{1.7 \ \cancel{M^2}} \times 25 \text{ mg} = 0.22 \times 25 \text{ mg} = 5.5 \text{ mg}$

---

85. $\dfrac{0.75 \ \cancel{M^2}}{1.7 \ \cancel{M^2}} \times 50 \text{ mg} = 0.44 \times 50 \text{ mg} = 22 \text{ mg}$

VI

Tools

☆ THIS SECTION CONTAINS TOOLS THAT WILL HELP you interpret physicians' medication orders, convert between different systems of measurement, and modify drug dosages for infants and children. You will also find an illustrated overview of medication forms.

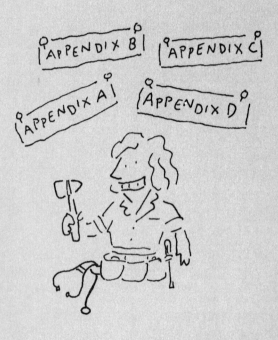

Abbreviations and Symbols

Physicians use abbreviations when prescribing medications. Knowledge of the meaning of abbreviations is necessary to interpret the written order correctly. For example, **Toradol 30 mg IM q.6h** means "Toradol 30 milligrams, intramuscular, every six hours." **Cytotec 200 mcg t.i.d. p.c. & h.s.** means "Cytotec 200 micrograms three times per day after meals and at hour of sleep." **ASA gr X q.4h p.r.n. if temp > 101 F°** means "Aspirin grains ten every four hours as necessary if temperature is greater than one hundred and one degrees Fahrenheit." Use the common abbreviations listed below to interpret orders found throughout this book.

Common Abbreviations

ā	before
a.c.	before meals
ad. lib.	as desired, freely
a.m.	morning
aq.	aqueous, water
b.i.d.	twice a day
c̄	with
D/C	discontinue
dr or ʒ	dram
D5W	5% dextrose in water
Dx	diagnosis
elix	elixir
g (Gm, gm)	gram
gr	grain
gtt	drop
h	hour
h.s.	hour of sleep
ID	intradermal
IM	intramuscular
IV	intravenous
IVPB	intravenous piggyback
kg	kilogram
K.V.O. (TKO)	keep vein open
L	liter

♏	minim
mcg	microgram
mEq	milliequivalent
mg (mgm)	milligram
mL (ml)	milliliter
NPO	nothing by mouth
NSS	normal saline solution
q.d.	every day
O.D.	right eye
O.S.	left eye
O.U.	both eyes
oz or ℥	ounce
p̄	after
p.c.	after meals
p.m.	afternoon, evening
p.o. (per os)	by mouth
p.r.n.	as needed
pt	pint
Pt.	patient
q	every
q.d.	every day
q.h.	every hour
q.2h	every two hours
q.4h	every four hours
q.6h	every six hours
q.8h	every eight hours
q.12h	every twelve hours
q.i.d.	four times a day
q.o.d.	every other day
q.s.	quantities sufficient
qt	quart
R/O	rule out
s̄	without
SC or SQ	subcutaneous
SL	sublingual
ss	one half
stat	immediately
supp	suppository
susp	suspension
tab(s)	tablet(s)
tbs or T	tablespoon
t.i.d.	three times a day
tsp or t	teaspoon
U	unit
>	greater than
<	less than

Preparation Forms and Packaging

Preparation Forms

Pharmaceutical companies manufacture medications in various preparation forms. Use this list of common preparation forms and definitions as a reference when interpreting medication orders.

1. **Aqueous solution:** one or more medications completely dissolved in water.

2. **Capsule:** gelatinous container enclosing a powder, a liquid, or time-release granules of medication.

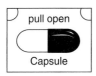 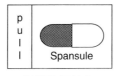

FIGURE B.1

3. **Elixir:** medication dissolved in a mixture of water, alcohol, sweeteners, and flavoring.

4. **Metered-dose inhaler:** aerosol device containing multiple doses of medication for inhalation.

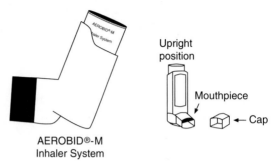

AEROBID®-M
Inhaler System

FIGURE B.2

5. **Ointment:** semisolid preparation of medication to be applied to the skin.

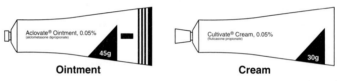

FIGURE B.3

6. **Suppository:** mixture of medication with a firm base that melts at body temperature and is molded into a shape suitable for insertion into body cavities.

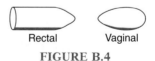

FIGURE B.4

7. **Suspension:** finely divided particles of medication undissolved in water.

8. **Syrup:** medication in water and sugar solution.

9. **Tablet:** powdered medication compressed or molded into a small disk.

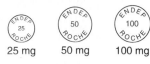

25 mg   50 mg   100 mg

FIGURE B.5

10. **Transdermal patch:** adhesive disk that attaches to the skin with a center reservoir containing medication to be slowly absorbed through the skin.

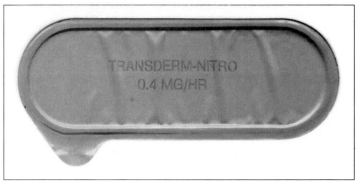

FIGURE B.6a

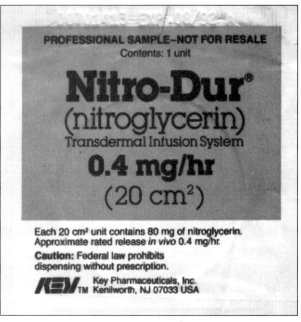

FIGURE B.6b

Catapres-TTS®-1
(clonidine)

Transdermal Therapeutic System

Programmed delivery *in vivo* of 0.1 mg per day for one week.

Boehringer Ingelheim

FIGURE B.6c

Transderm-Nitro®
(nitroglycerin)

Transdermal Therapeutic System

0.4 mg/hr

FOR TRANSDERMAL USE ONLY

Easy-to-Open Tab

Summit Pharmaceuticals
Division of CIBA–GEIGY Corporation

Summit Pharmaceuticals
Division of CIBA–GEIGY Corporation

Contents: 5 systems

Each 20 cm² system contains 50 mg nitroglycerin. The inactive components are lactose, silicone medical fluid, aluminized plastic, silicone medical adhesive, ethylene/vinyl acetate copolymer, and colloidal silicon dioxide.

Rated release *in vivo* 0.4 mg/hr

Dosage and Administration: Follow dosing instructions as directed by your physician. For application, see patient instructions.

Do not store above 86°F.

See bottom panel for lot

Transderm-Nitro®
(nitroglycerin)

FIGURE B.6d

Parenteral Packaging

There are three common types of parenteral medication containers for sterile solutions.

1. **Ampule:** sealed glass container with only one dose of powdered or liquid medication.

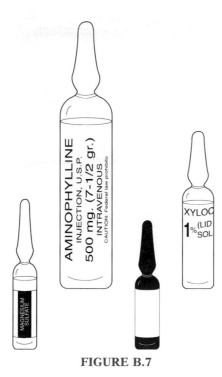

FIGURE B.7

2. **Prefilled cartridge:** small, slender single-dose vial with an attached needle. A metal or plastic holder is used to inject the medication.

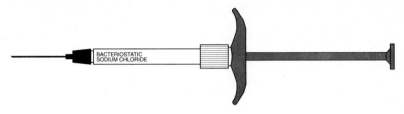

Prefilled cartridge and holder

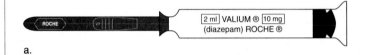

a.

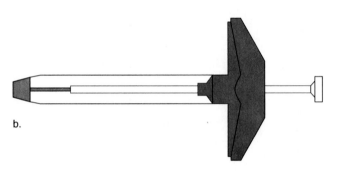

b.

a. Prefilled cartridge
b. Cartridge holder

FIGURE B.8

3. **Vial:** sealed glass container of a liquid or powdered medication with a rubber stopper, allowing multiple dose use.

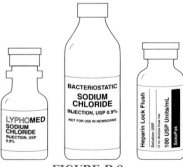

FIGURE B.9

Clark's, Fried's, and Young's Rules for Pediatric Dosage Computations

Three less frequently used methods for calculating pediatric drug dosages are Clark's, Fried's and Young's rules. Using these methods will provide only a ROUGH estimate of pediatric dosages. Use them only in an emergency situation when lack of information prevents the use of the dosage-per-kilogram-of-body-weight and body-surface-area methods.

CLARK'S RULE

(Based on infant/child weight in pounds
and the average adult weight of 150 pounds)

Formula: $\dfrac{\text{child's wt in lbs}}{150 \text{ lbs}} \times \text{normal adult dose} = \text{child's dose}$

Example: Child's weight = 40 lbs

Average Adult Dose of Keflex = 500 mg p.o. q.i.d.

$$\frac{40 \text{ lb}}{150 \text{ lb}} \times \frac{500 \text{ mg}}{1} = \frac{2000 \text{ mg}}{15} = 133 \text{ mg (child's dose)}$$

FRIED'S RULE

(For children from birth to 2 years old)

Formula: $\dfrac{\text{age in months}}{150} \times \text{normal adult dose} = \text{child's dose}$

Example: Child's age = 18 months

Average Adult Dose = FeSO4 325 mg p.o. b.i.d.

$$\frac{18 \text{ months}}{150 \text{ months}} \times \frac{325 \text{ mg}}{1} = 0.12 \times 325 \text{ mg} = 39 \text{ mg}$$

(child's dose)

YOUNG'S RULE

(For children 2 to 12 years of age)

Formula: $\dfrac{\text{age in years}}{\text{age in years} + 12} \times \text{normal adult dose} = \dfrac{\text{child's}}{\text{dose}}$

Example: Child's age = 8 years

Average Adult Dose = Demerol 75 mg IM q.4h
p.r.n. pain

$$\frac{8}{20} \times \frac{75 \text{ mg}}{1} = 0.4 \times 75 \text{ mg} = 30 \text{ mg}$$

Celsius and Fahrenheit Temperatures

Measuring a patient's temperature is probably one of the most basic procedures performed. Most hospitals and other health care settings use the Fahrenheit (F) temperature scale. However, there is an increasing tendency to use the Celsius or centigrade (C) temperature scale. Although equivalency tables are available, it is important to know how to convert between the two scales.*

Common Equivalents

Freezing	0° C	32° F
Normal Body Temperature	37° C	98.6° F
Boiling Point of Water	100° C	212° F

Conversion Formulas

Formula 1   Fahrenheit to Celsius
$$C = (F - 32)(0.555)$$

Example: F = 103°   C = ?
$$C = (103 - 32)(0.555)$$
$$C = (71)(0.555)$$
$$C = 39.405$$
$$C = 39.4°$$

Formula 2   Celsius to Fahrenheit
$$F = (C)(1.8) + 32$$

Example: C = 39°   F = ?
$$F = (39)(1.8) + 32$$
$$F = 70.2 + 32$$
$$F = 102.2°$$

*NOTE: Temperatures are rounded to the nearest tenth.

Notes

Notes

Notes

Notes

Notes

Notes

Notes

Notes

Notes

Notes

Notes